Getting Ready for™ My Blood Test

A Blood Test Book for Kids - Preparation and Recovery

AF688363

This book belongs to:

Written by Dr. Fei Zheng-Ward Illustrated by Moch. Fajar Shobaru

Identifiers: ISBN 979-8-89318-200-2 (eBook)
ISBN 979-8-89318-201-9 (paperback)
ISBN 979-8-89318-202-6 (hardcover)

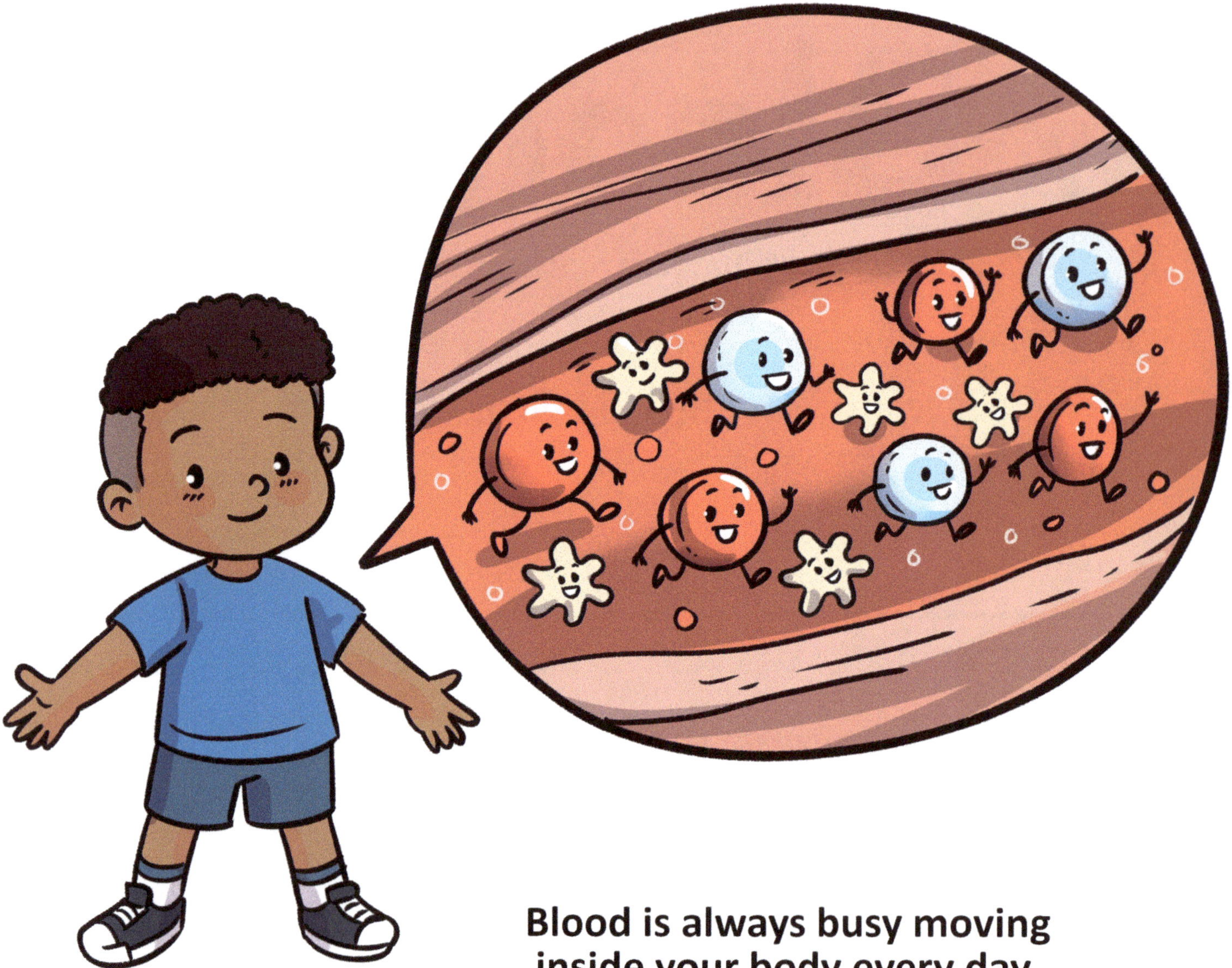

Blood is always busy moving inside your body every day.

Everyone needs a blood test sometimes.

A blood test is when a medical helper takes a little bit of your blood to learn important things about your body.

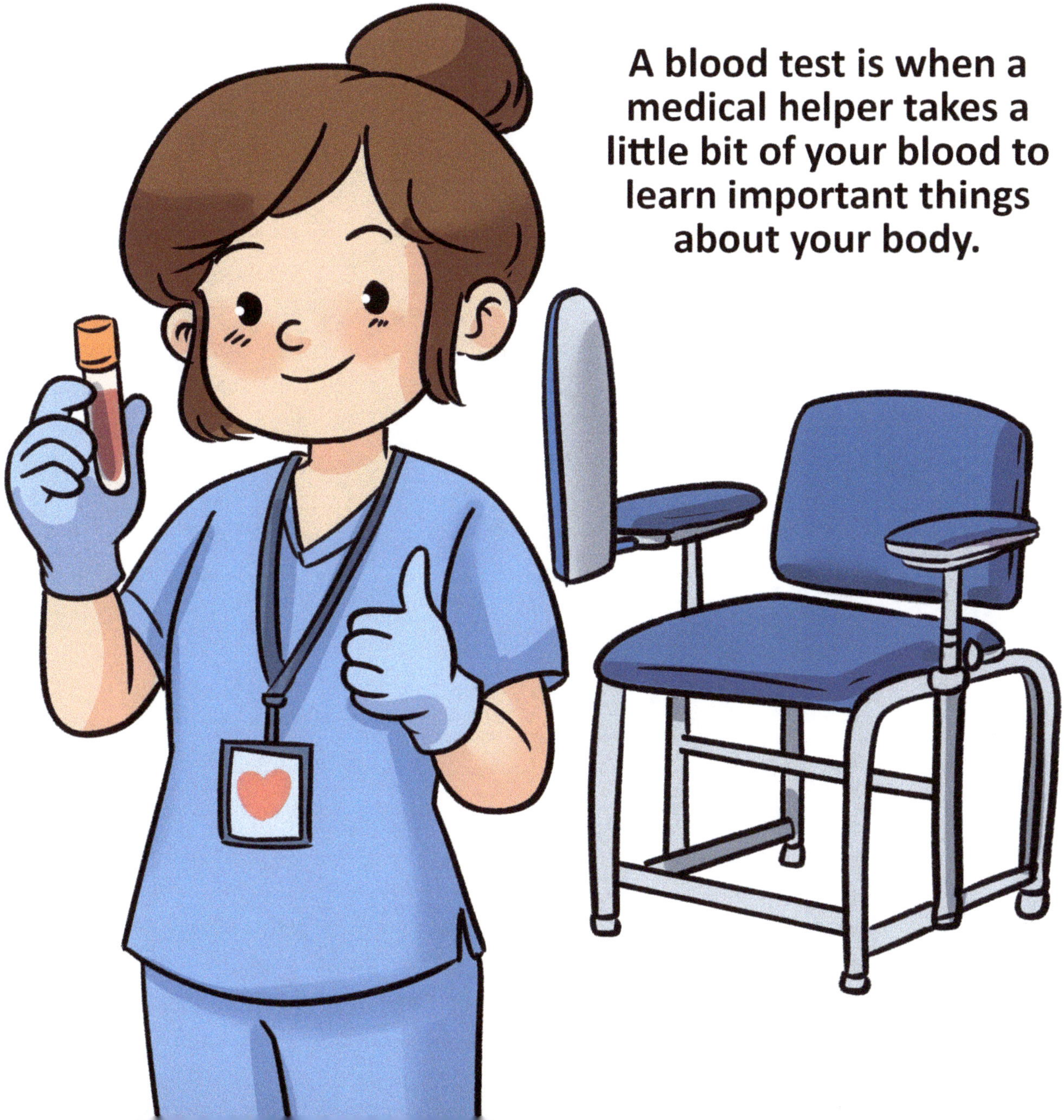

Blood carries oxygen to different parts of your body so you can do all the things you love.

It carries nutrients to help your body grow and tiny helpers that fight germs and help you heal.

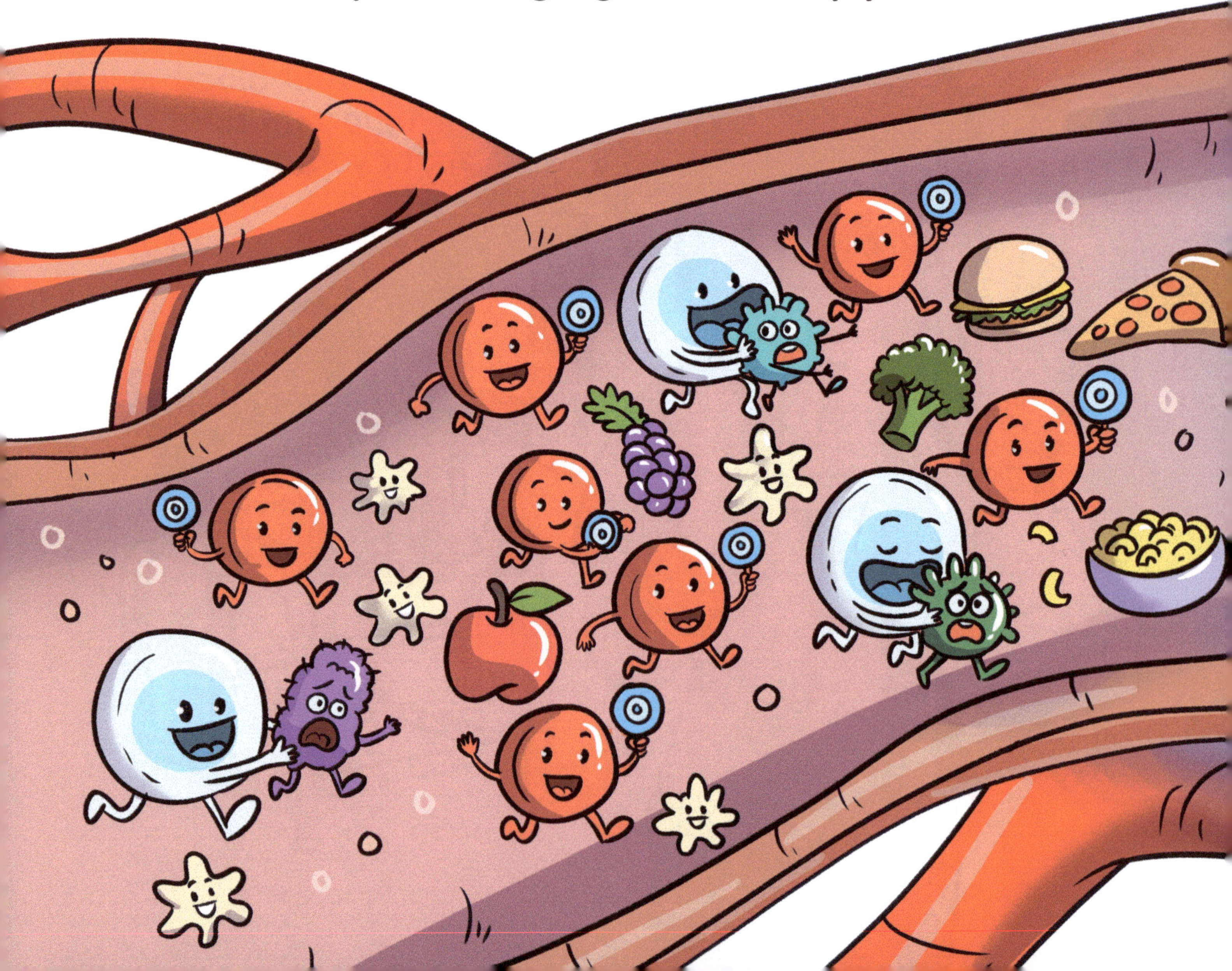

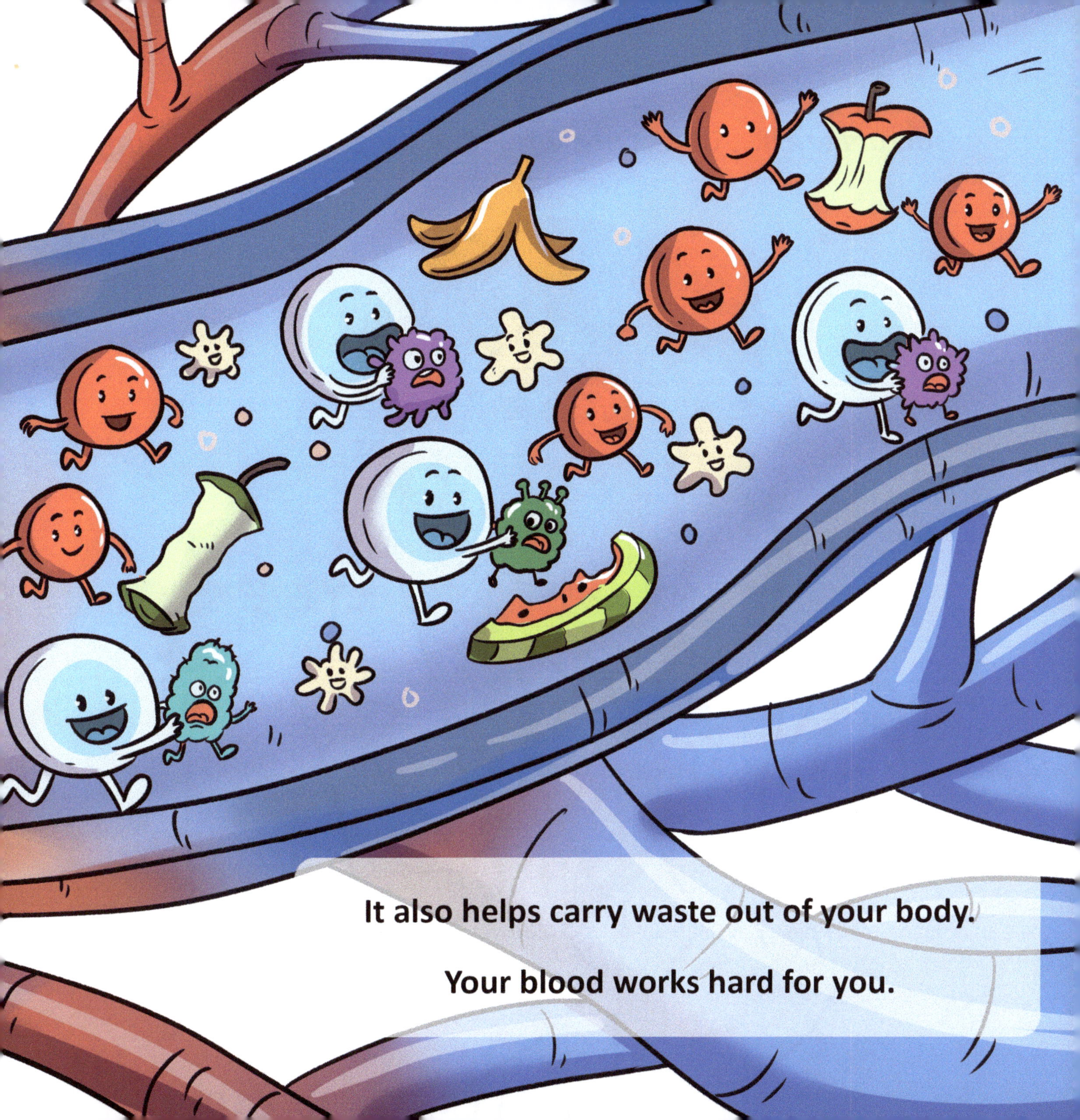

It also helps carry waste out of your body.

Your blood works hard for you.

Doctors are like detectives who look for clues in your blood.

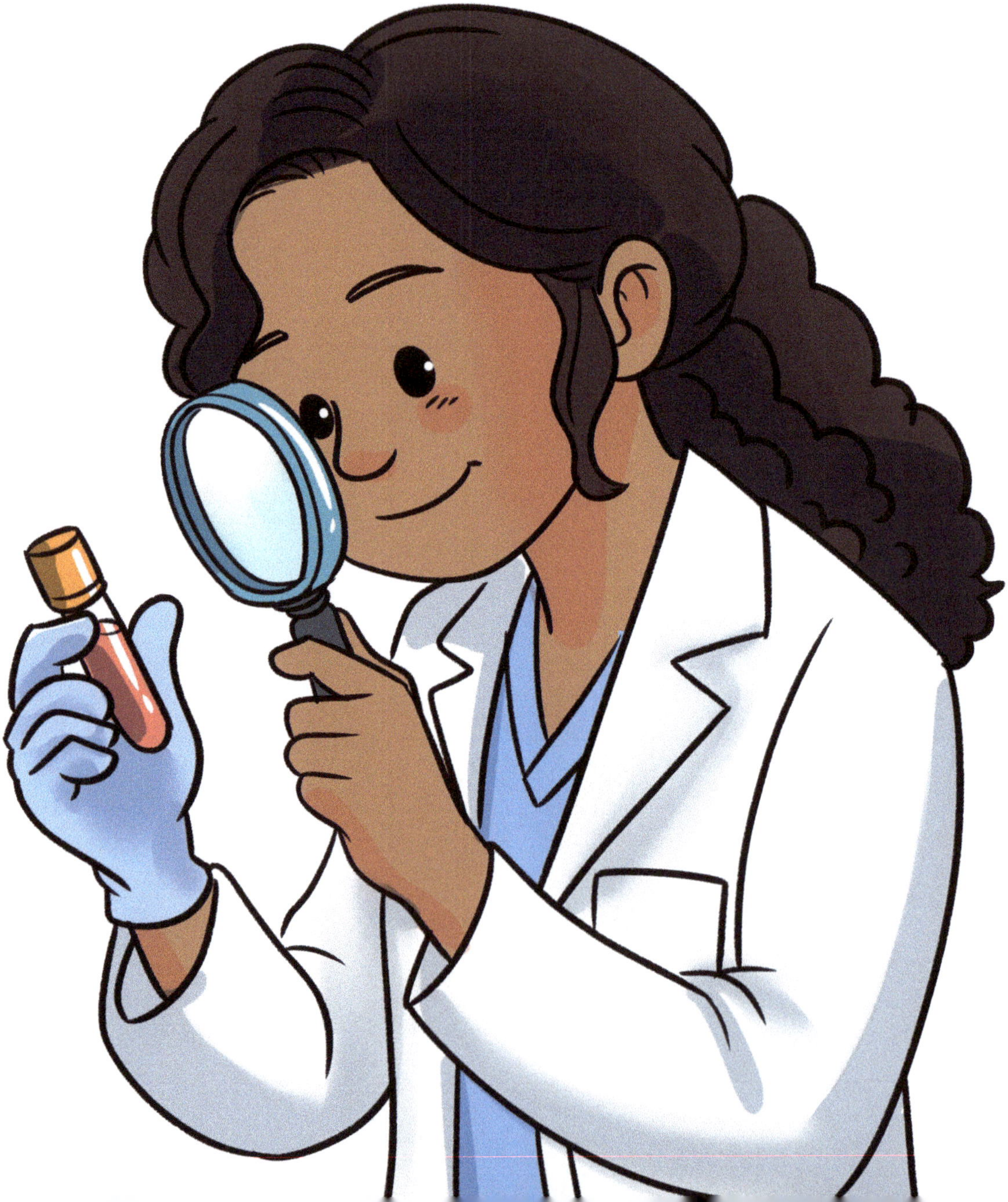

A blood test gives important clues to

☐ why someone is not feeling well

☐ how much sugar is in the blood

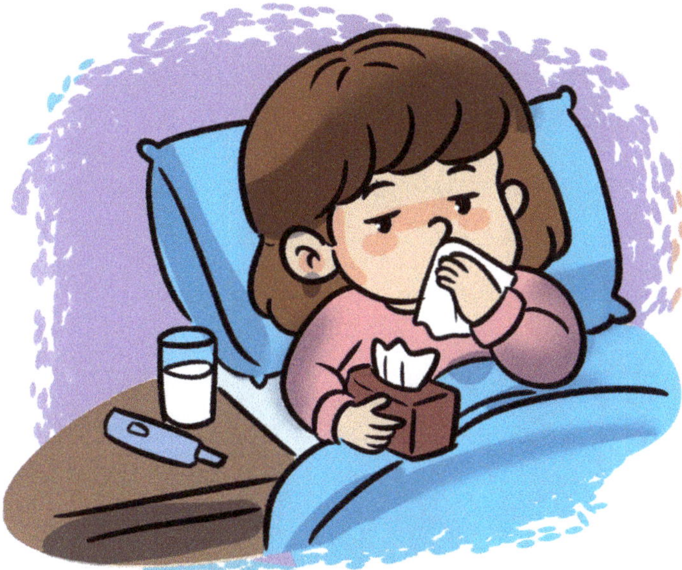

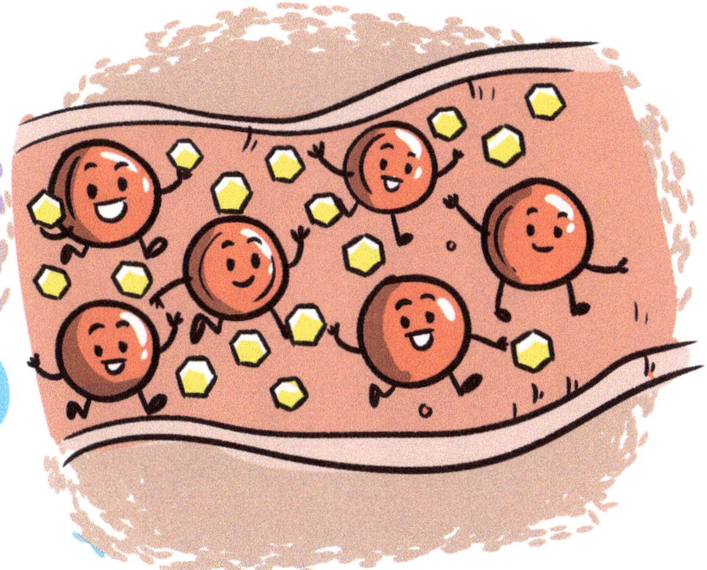

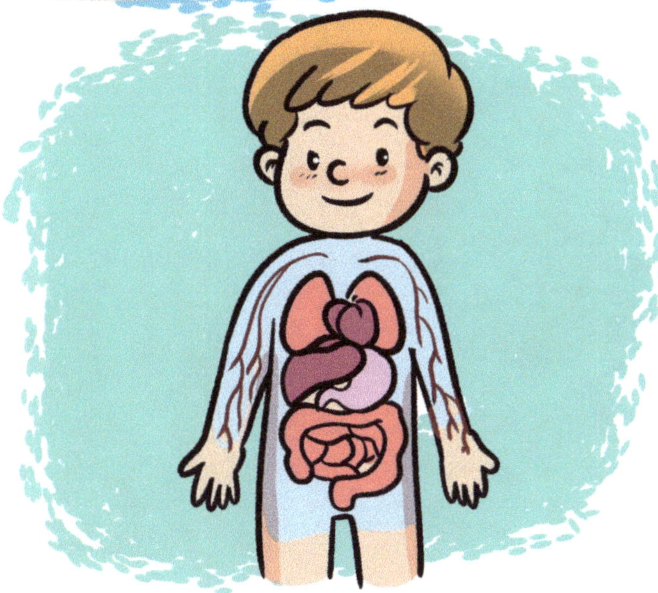

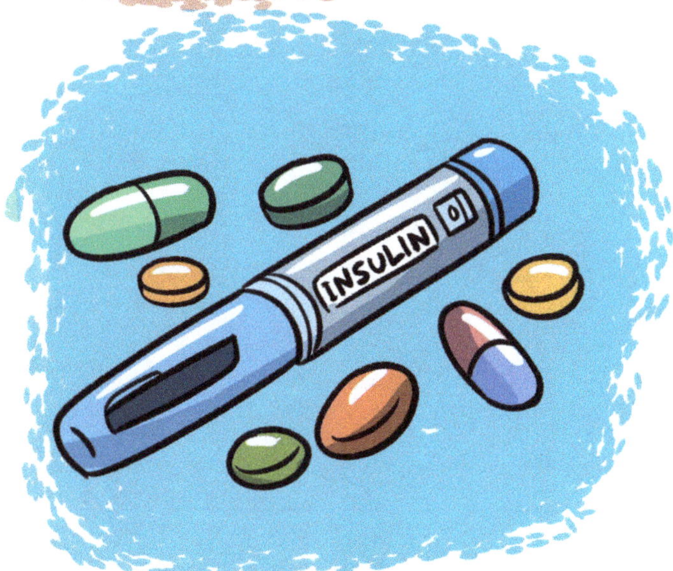

☐ how the body is working

☐ if medicine is helping someone get better

The doctor only needs a small amount,
like taking a little bite out of a big pizza.

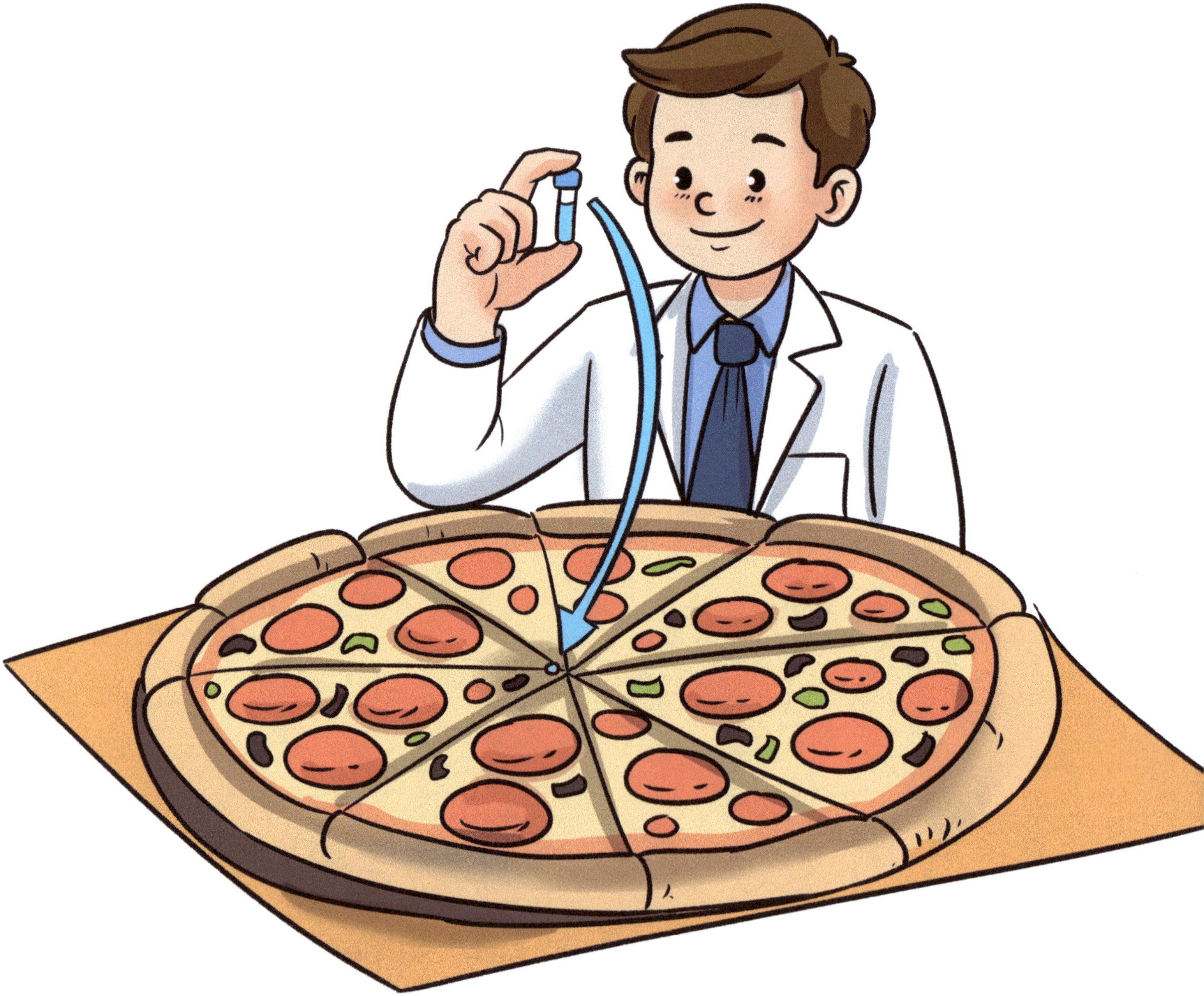

Your body has a lot more blood than the test needs.

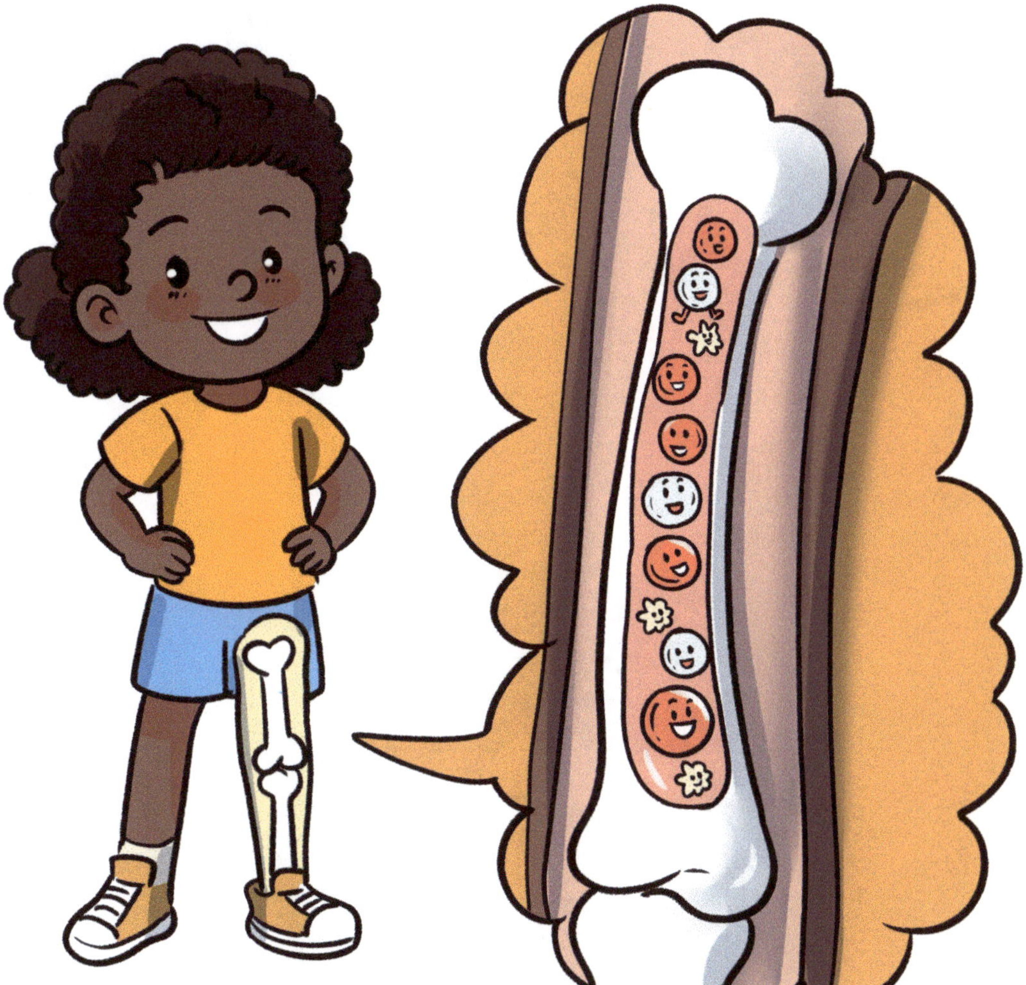

After the test, your body makes more blood on its own.
That's something your body is good at.

You may feel

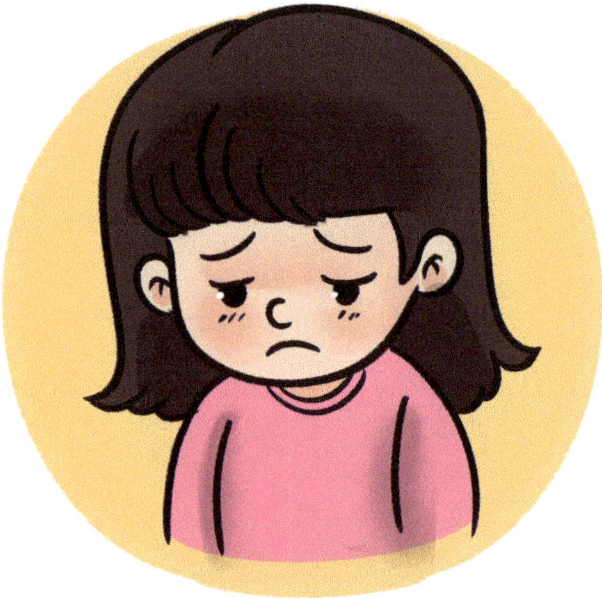

sad

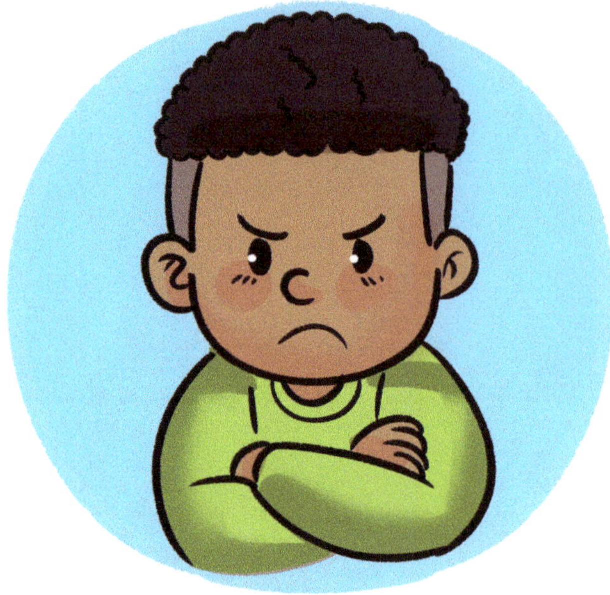

mad

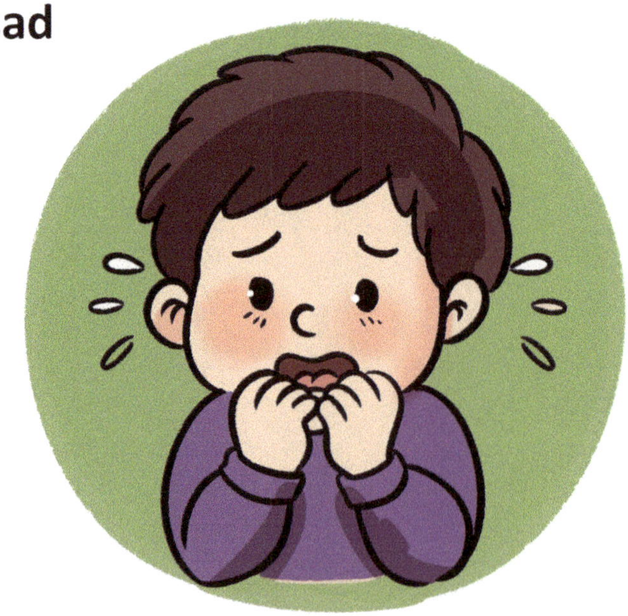

scared

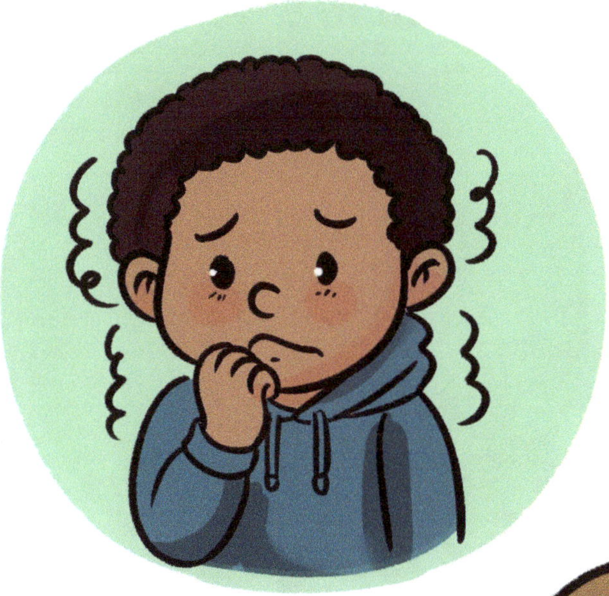

nervous

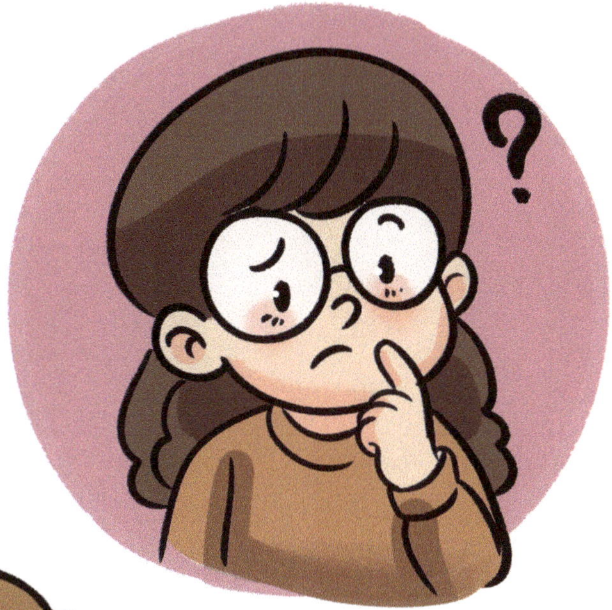

confused

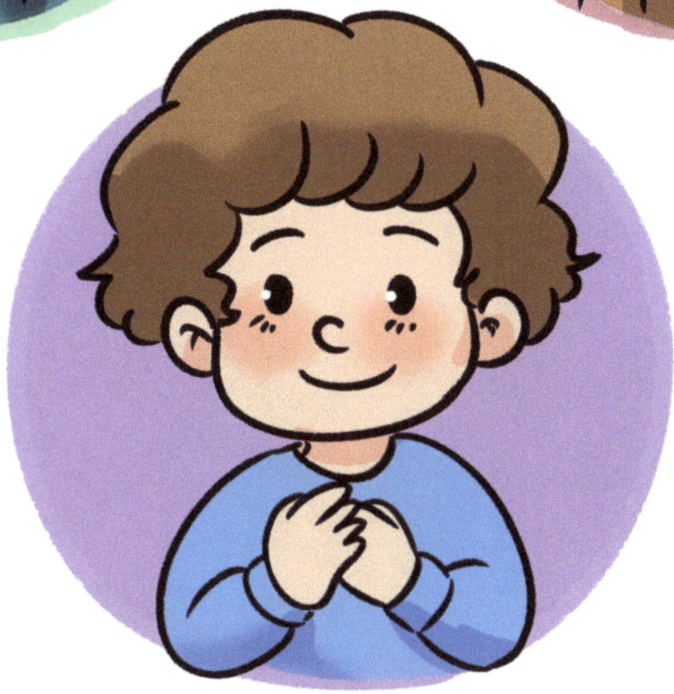

I can do my best!

Or, you might not know how you feel yet.
However you feel today is okay.

Some blood tests need an empty tummy,
and some do not.

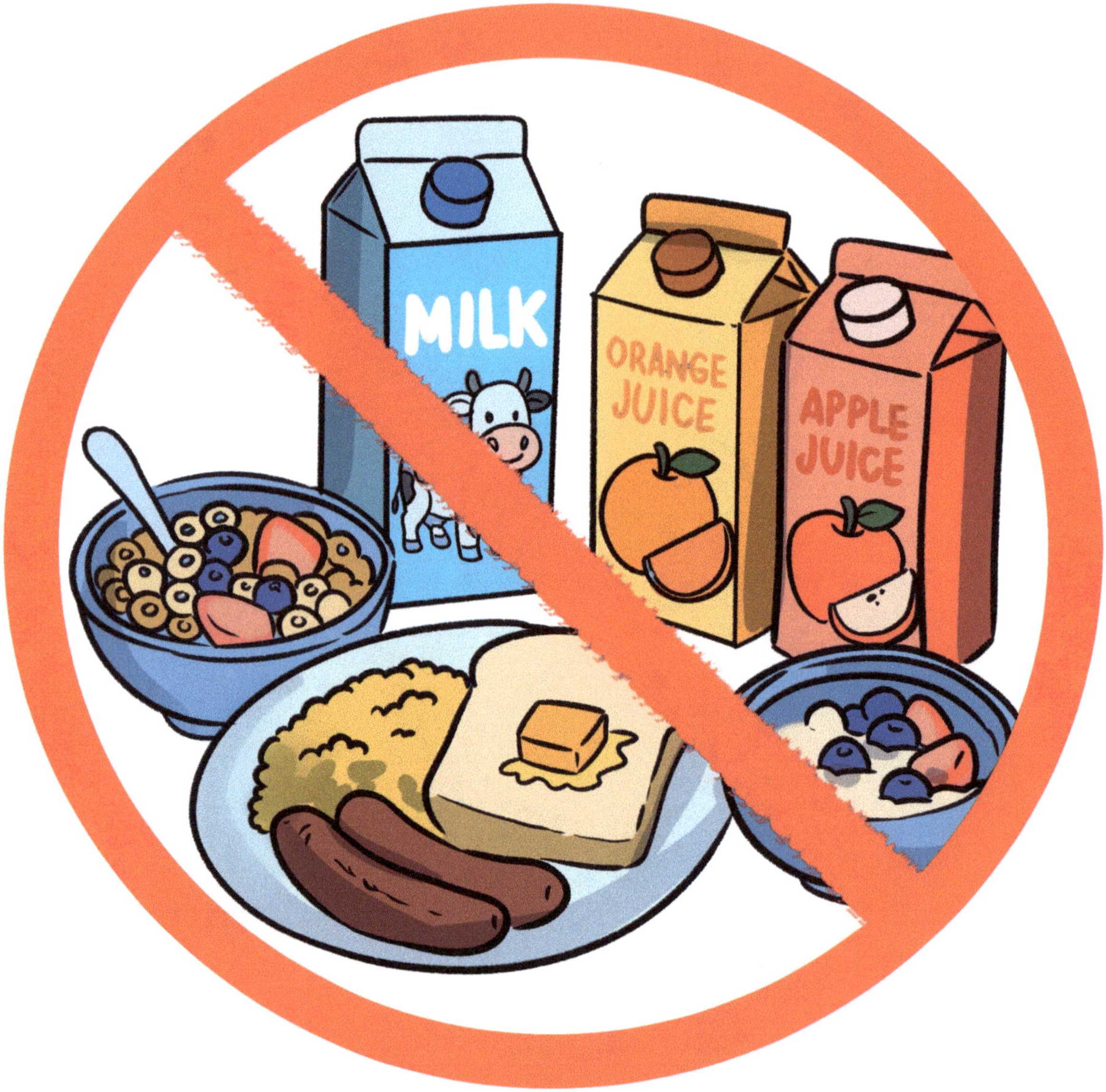

Your doctor and grown-up will let you know.

You'll meet a special medical helper who collects blood.
This helper is called a phlebotomist.

Their job is to collect blood safely and carefully.

They do this every day and for many kids just like you.

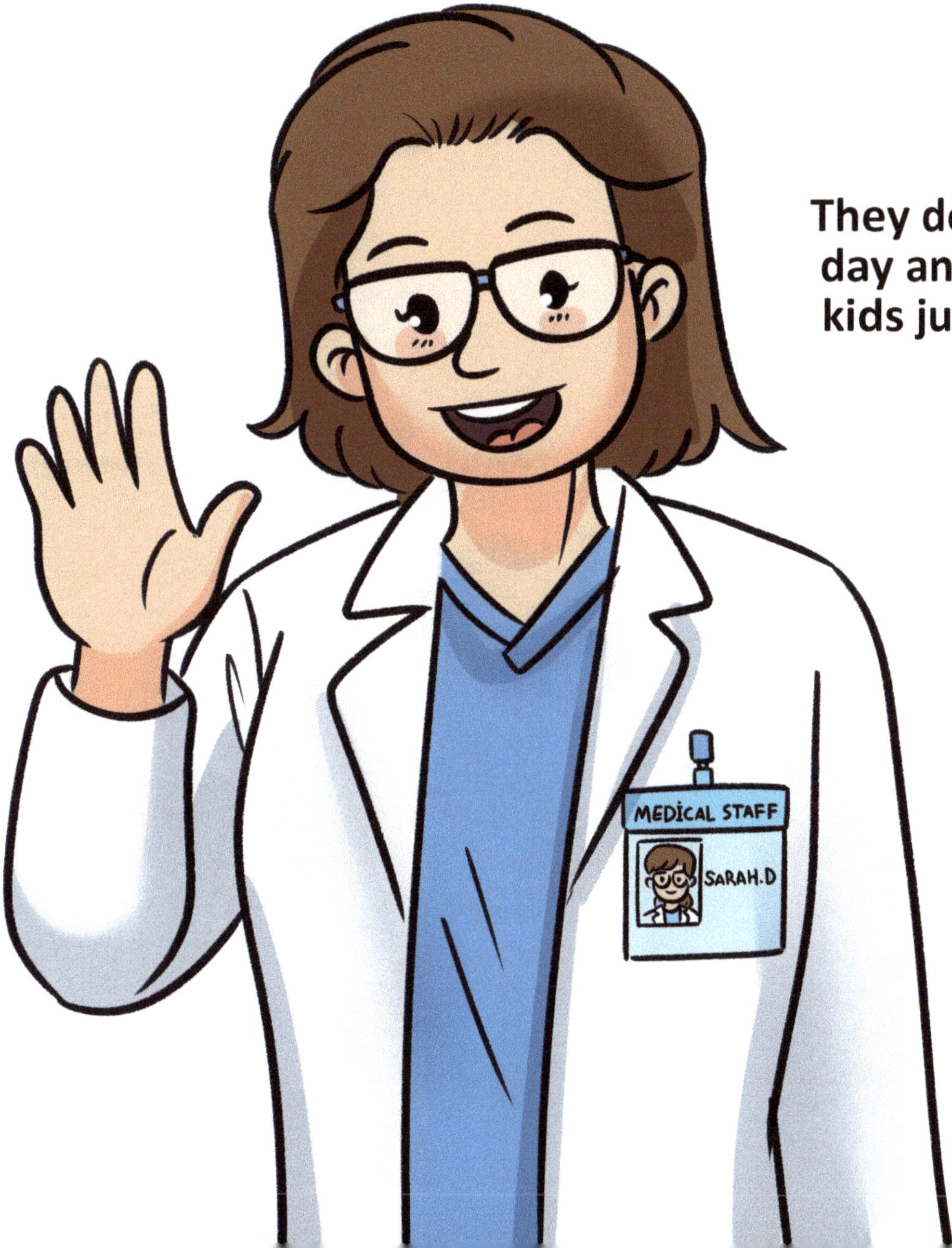

They may ask for your name and birthday
and why you're there.

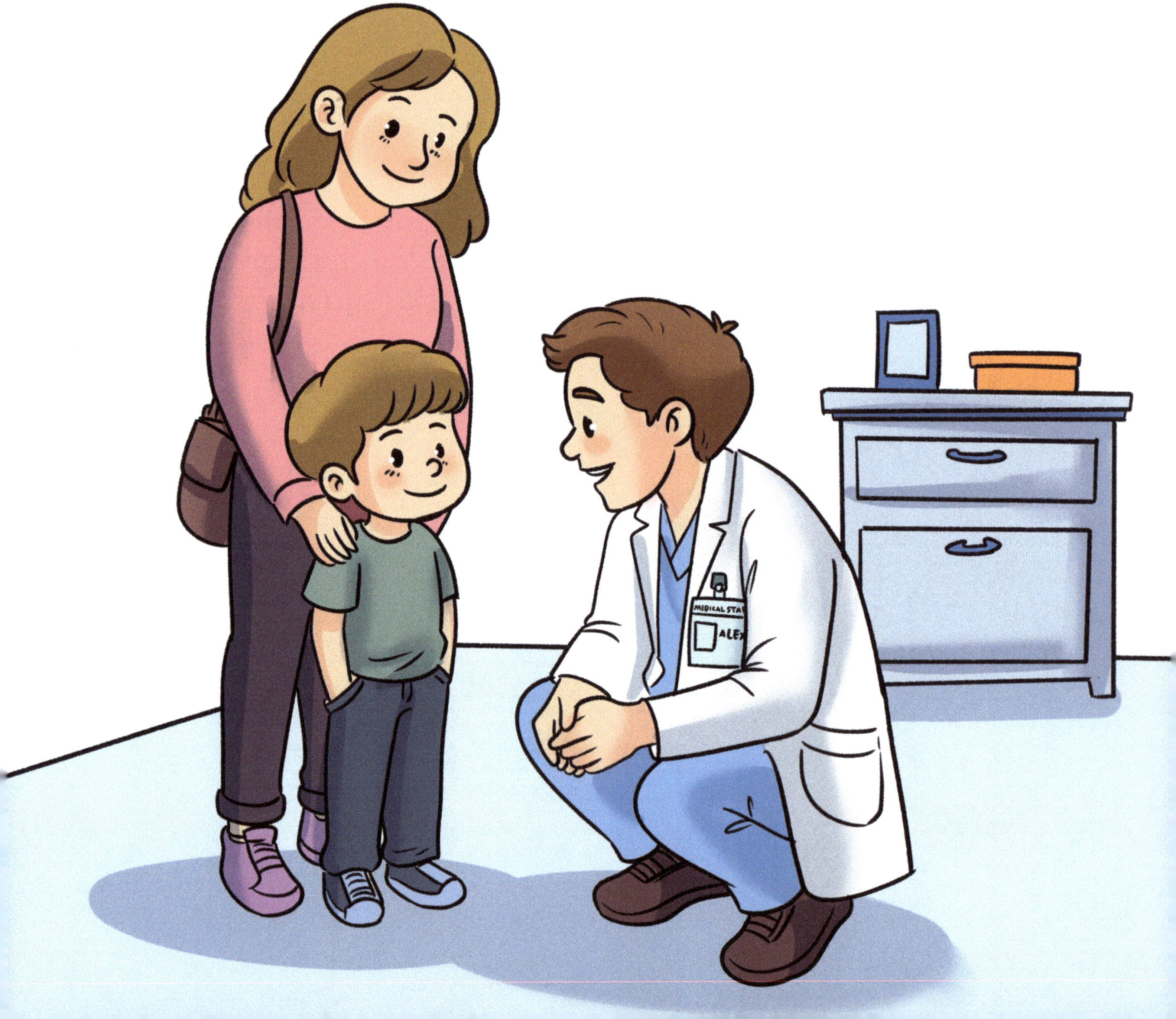

If you have any questions, feel free to ask.
Everyone is here to help you.

You've got this!

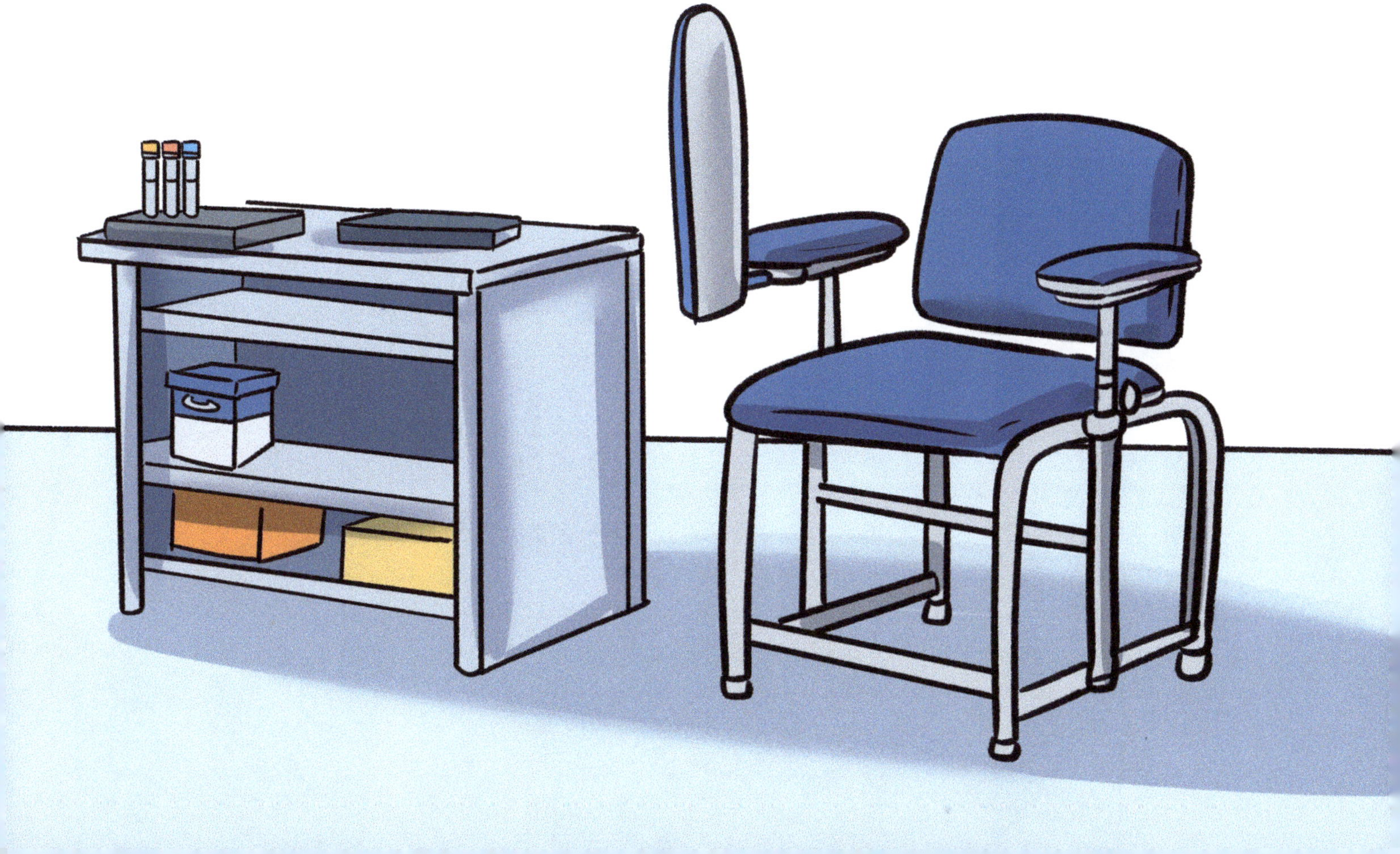

You may sit in a special chair or on a grown-up's lap.

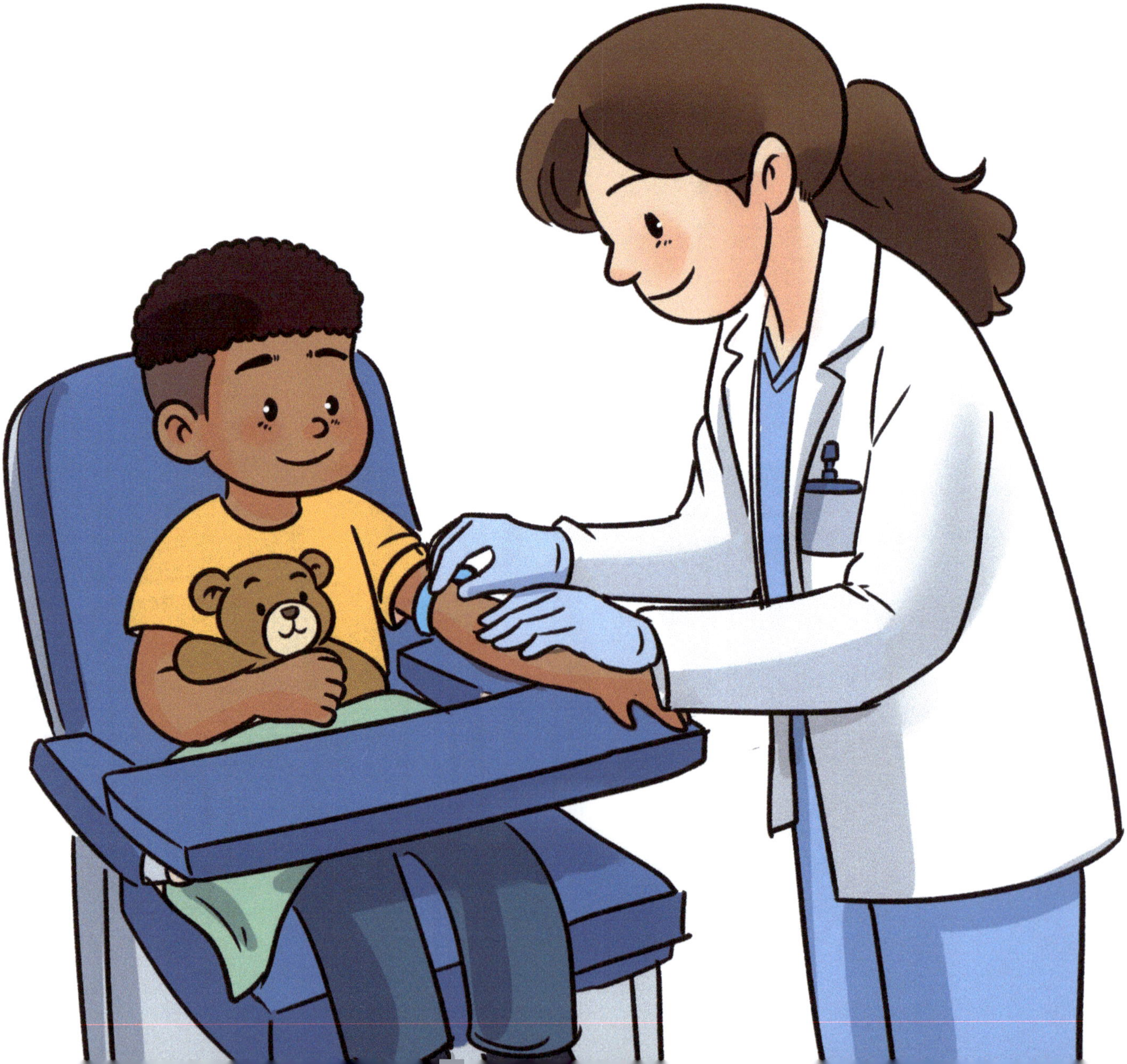

Your grown-up will stay with you the whole time.

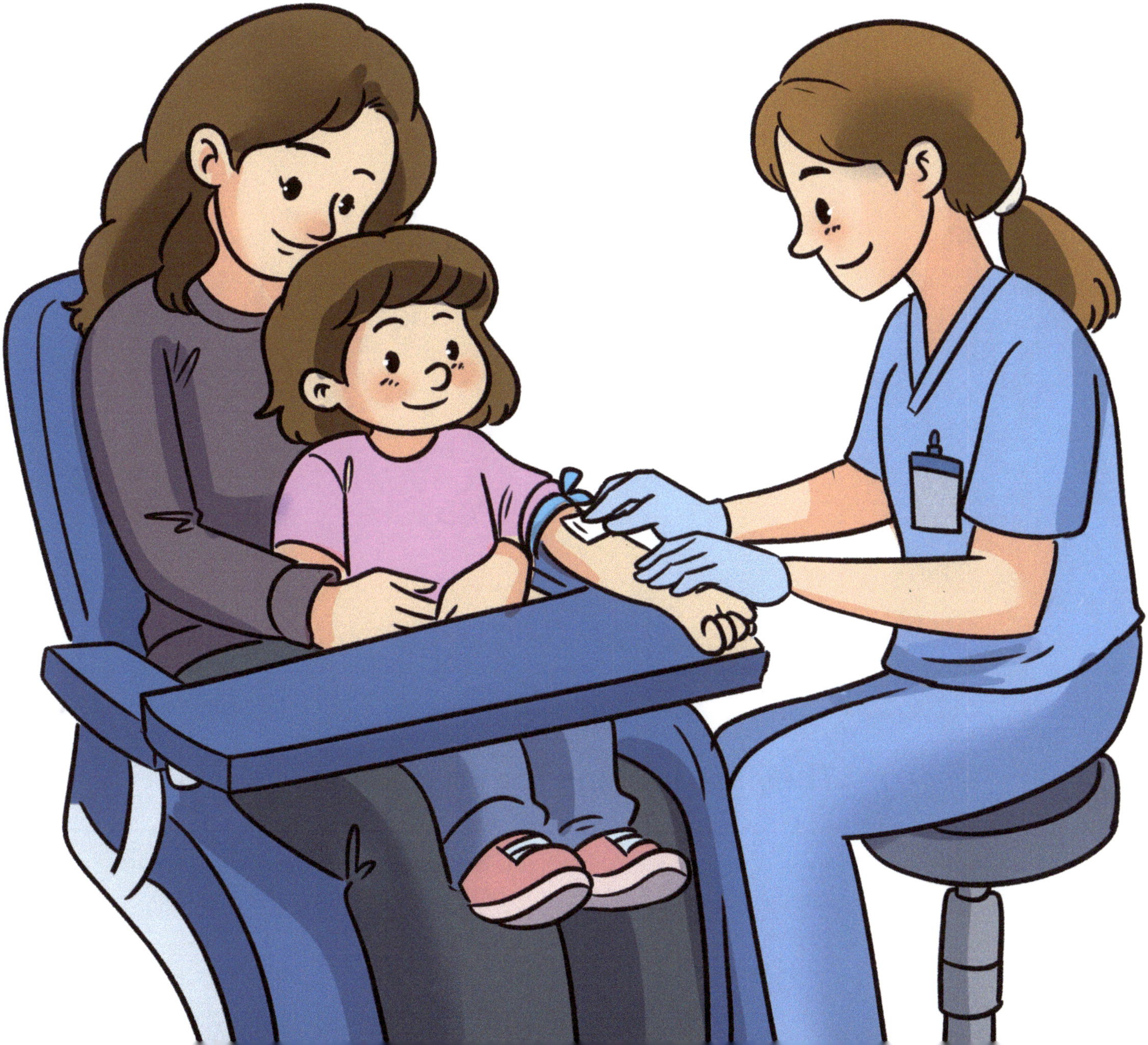

The medical helper may look at your hands, arms, and sometimes even your feet.

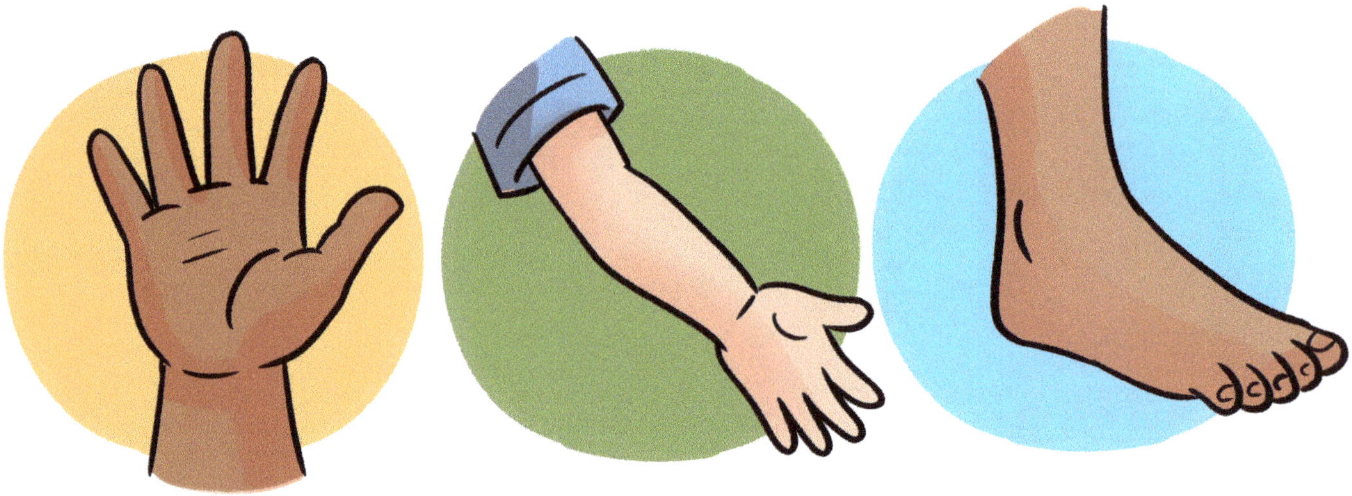

They are looking for your veins.

Veins are small long tunnels under your skin that carry blood around your body.

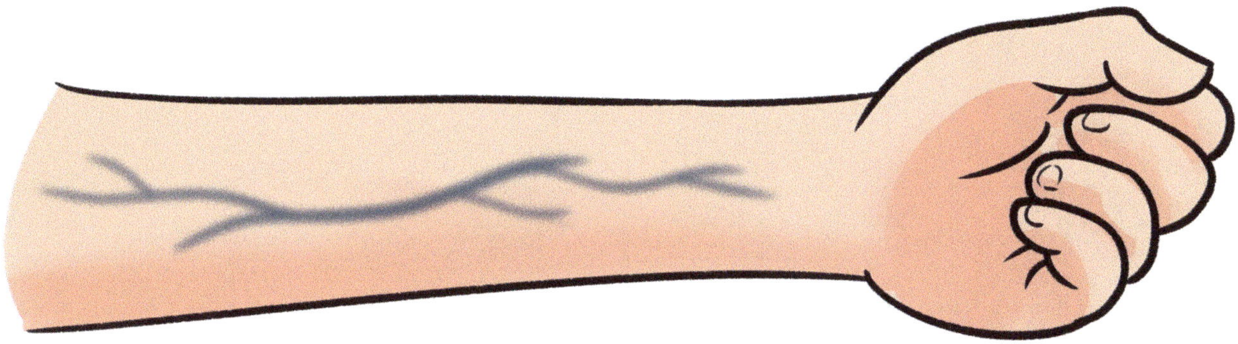

You can sometimes see your veins.

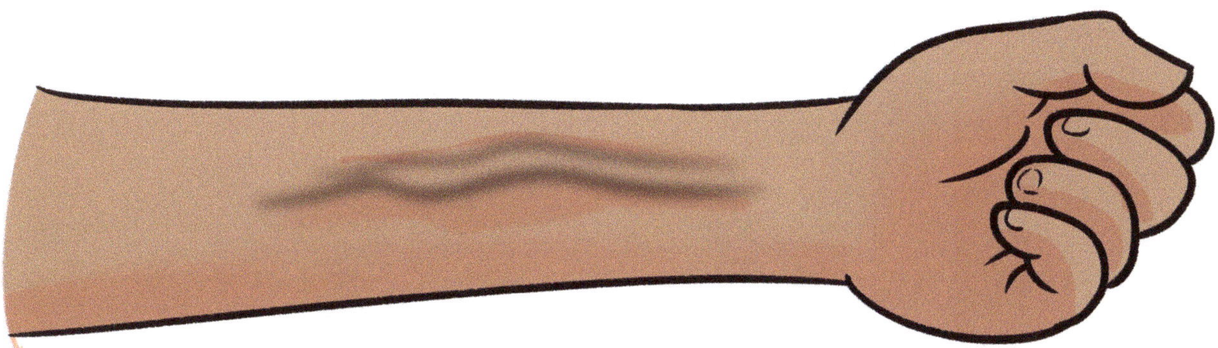

They can look like bluish or little squishy tunnels under your skin.

First, a stretchy band goes around your arm and can feel tight.
The band helps make your veins easier to see.

The stretchy bands come in different colors. What color will yours be?

Red Green

Yellow Blue

Pink Orange

Purple

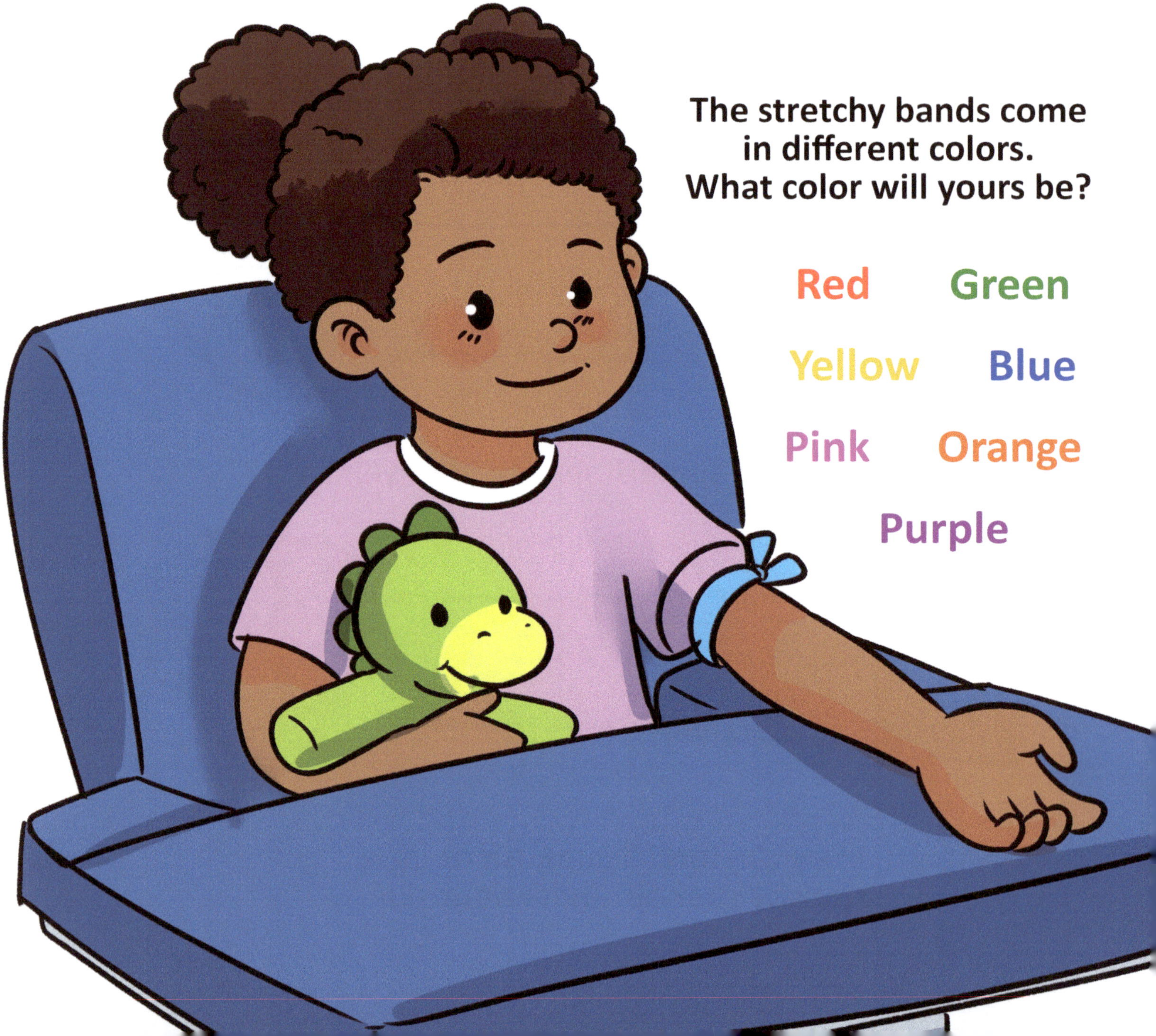

Did you know that if you open and close
your hand a few times that can also
help make your veins easier to see?

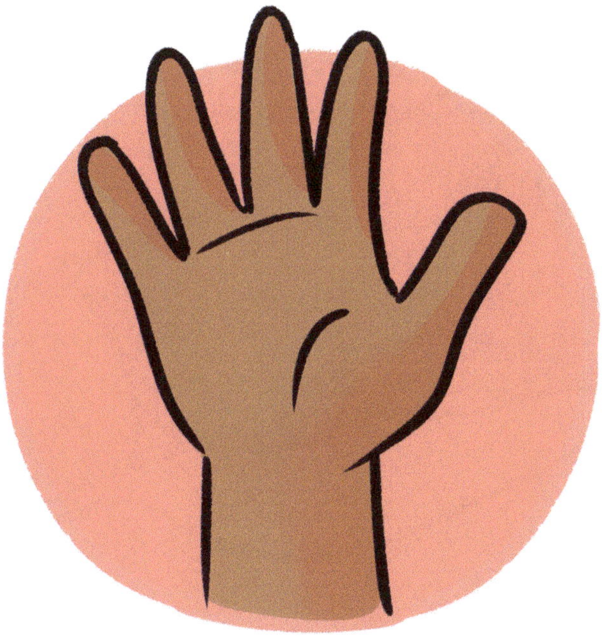

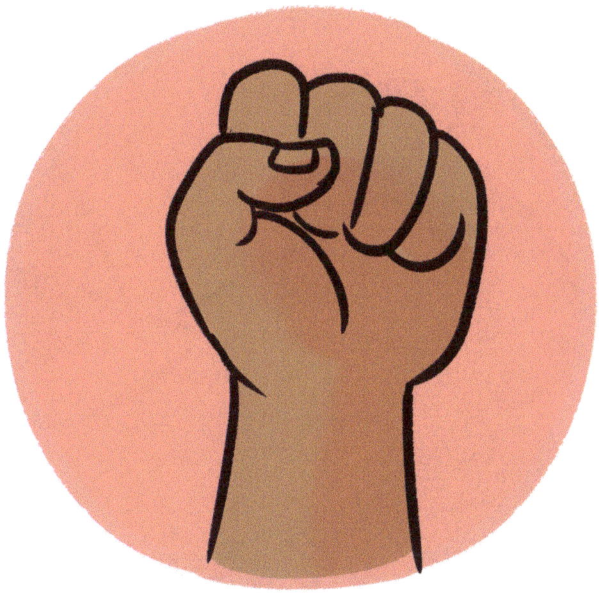

Let's practice opening and closing your hand
to get ready for your blood test.

You are so brave!

Next, your skin is cleaned with a small wipe.
It may feel cold and wet, and it may smell funny.

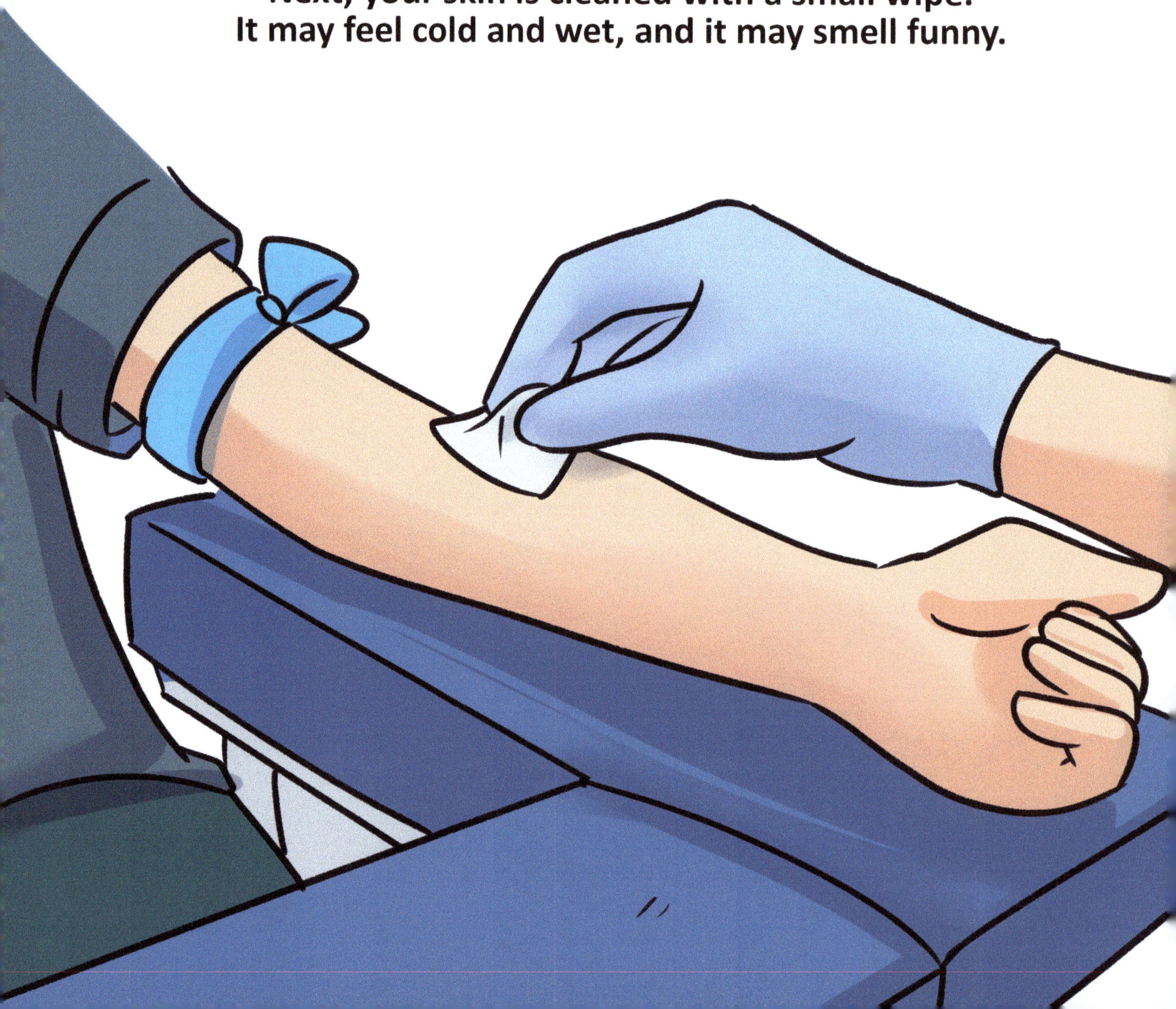

Then, you may feel a quick poke or pinch.

Did you know that some needles look like butterflies?
And, they come in different colors.
What color will yours be?

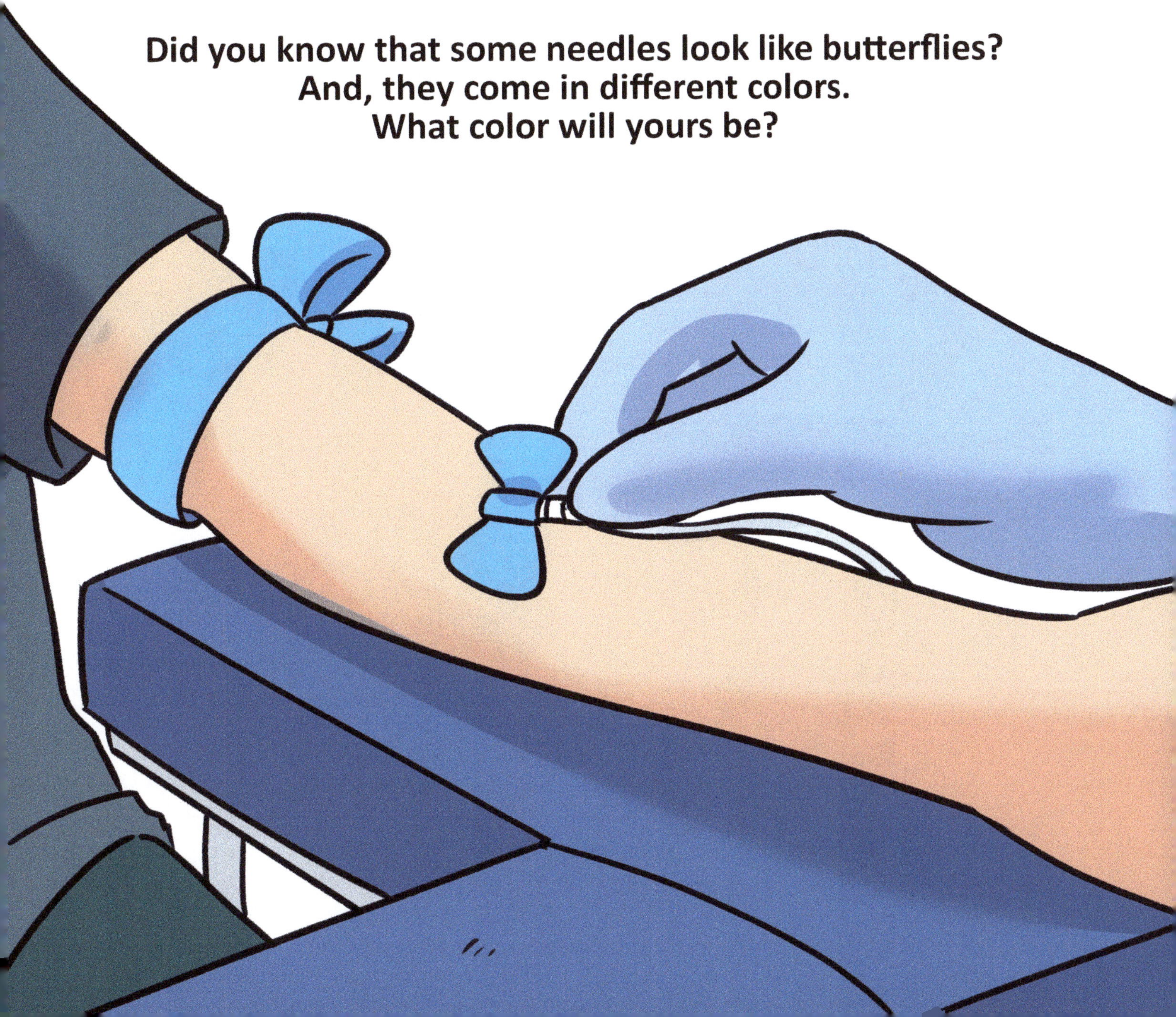

What do you want to do when they're drawing your blood?
Mark your favorites.

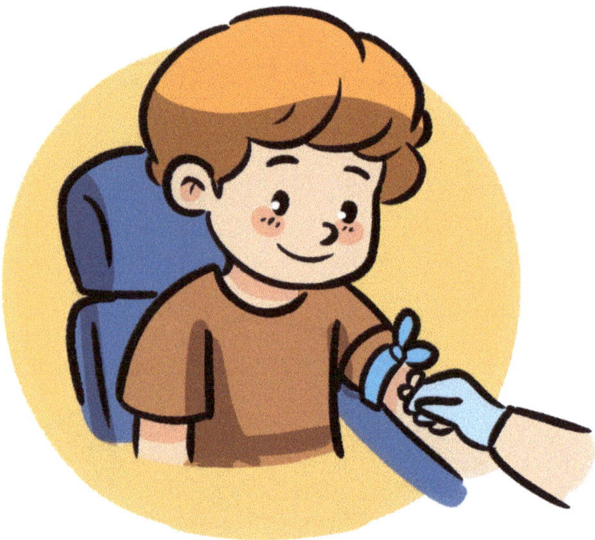

☐ Watch

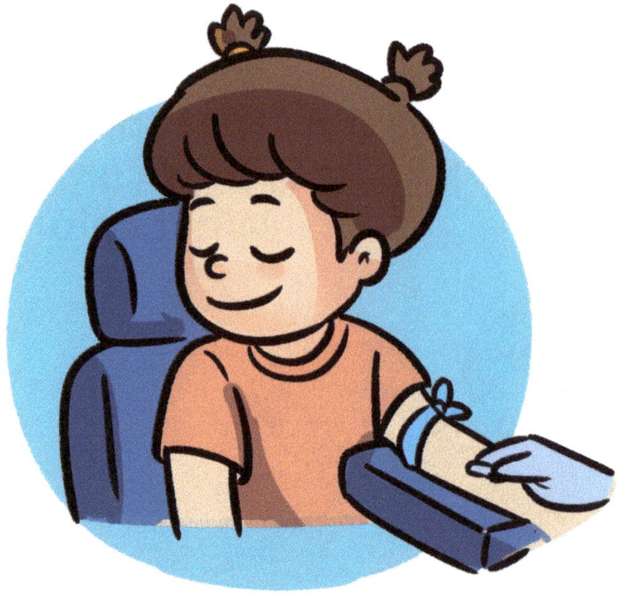

☐ Turn my head away

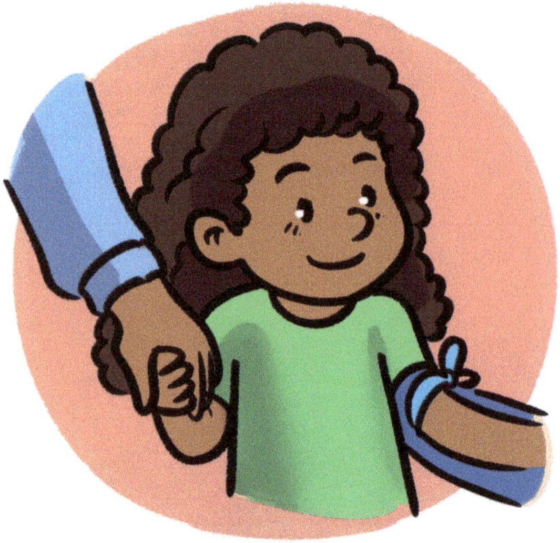

☐ Hold my parent or guardian's hand

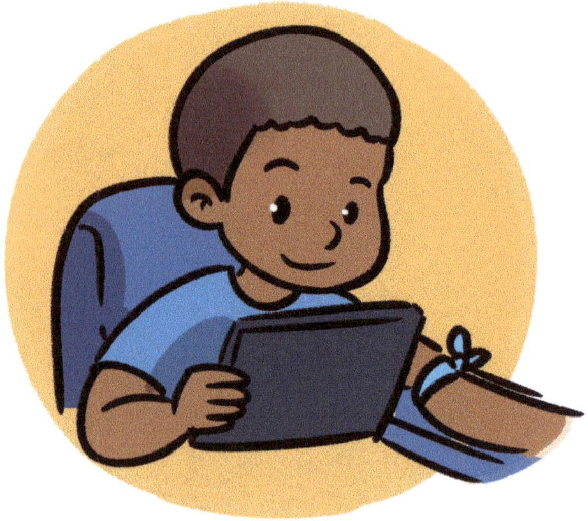

☐ Watch a video

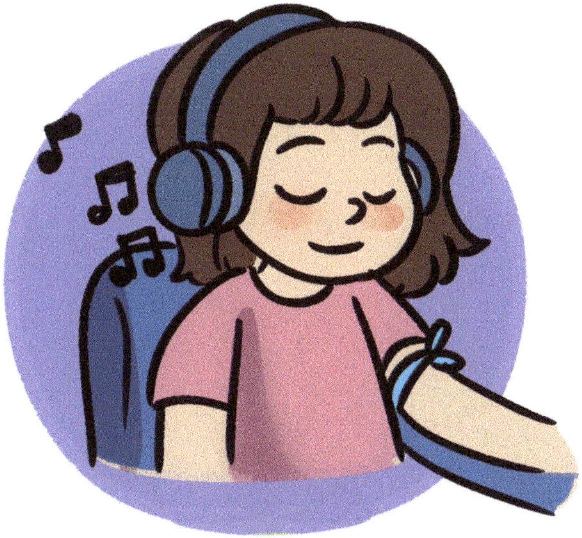

☐ Listen to music

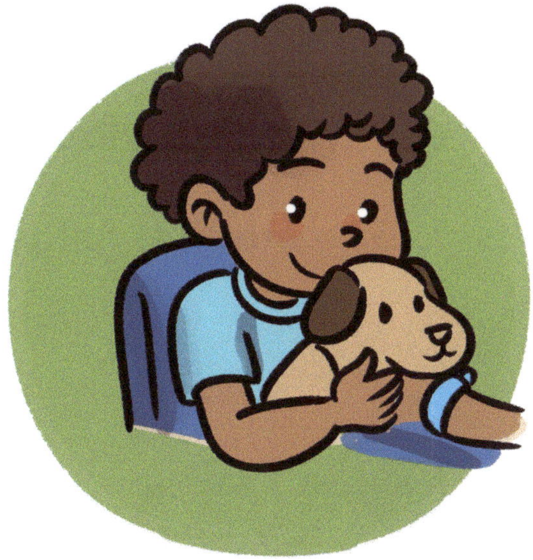

☐ Hold onto my favorite toy

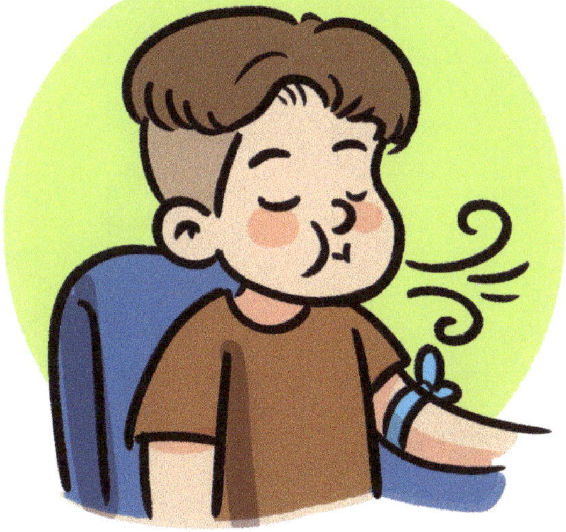

☐ Take slow belly breaths

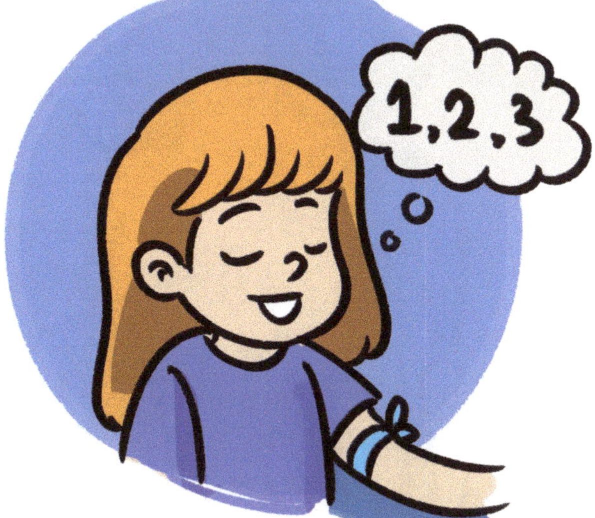

☐ Counting slowly

What creative ideas do you have?

Your blood flows into small tubes.

The medical helper may fill one or a few tubes.

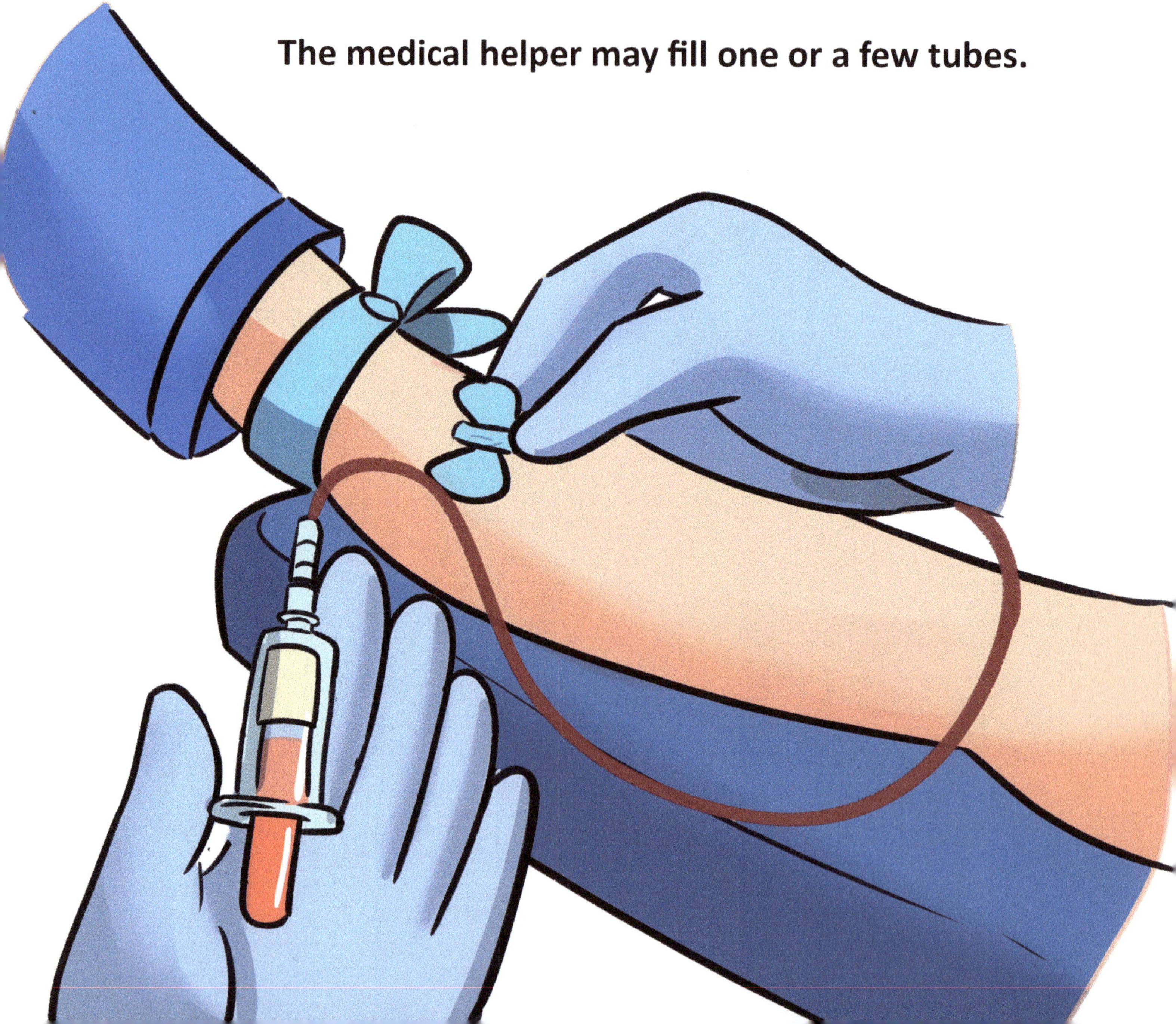

You can help by staying very still, like a statue
or a game of freeze, which do you prefer?

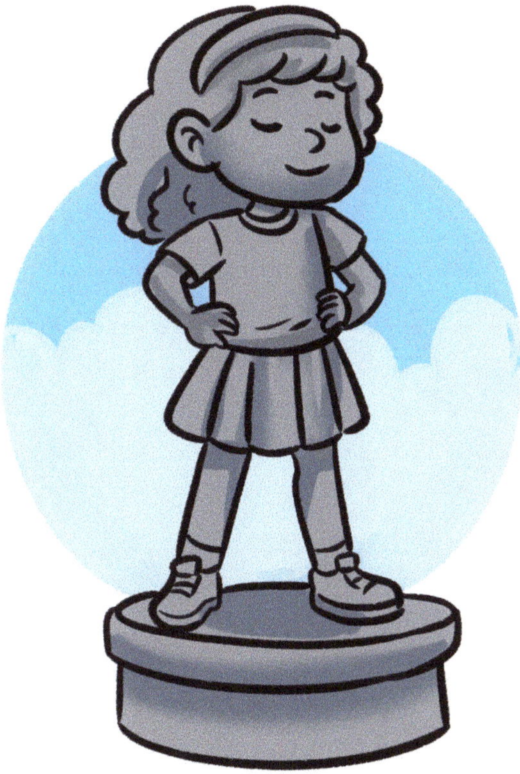

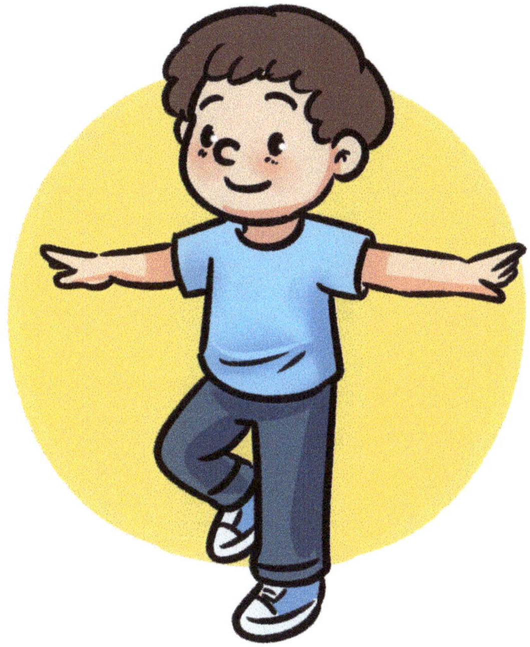

Staying still often helps the blood test go quicker.

If your body wiggles, that's okay.

The medical helper and your grown-up
will help you get steady again.

When the small tubes are full, the stretchy band comes off.

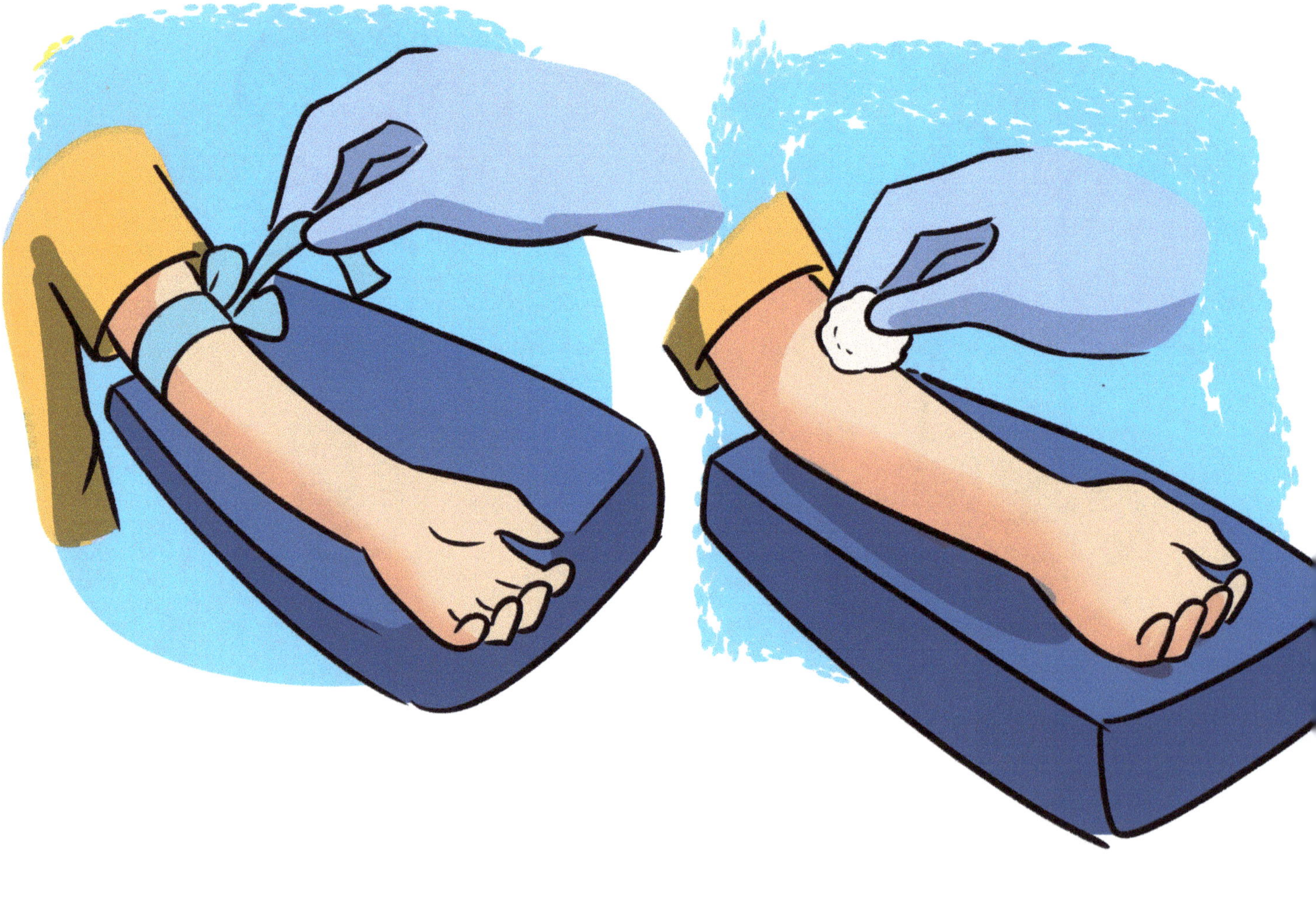

A soft cotton ball or gauze is pressed on the spot.

You may help to press and hold the cotton ball or gauze.

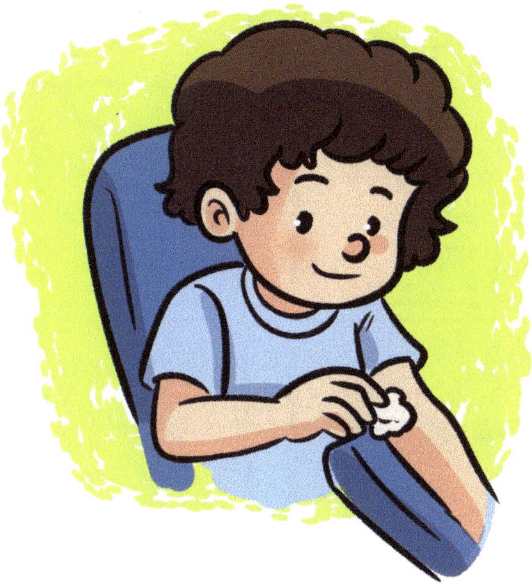

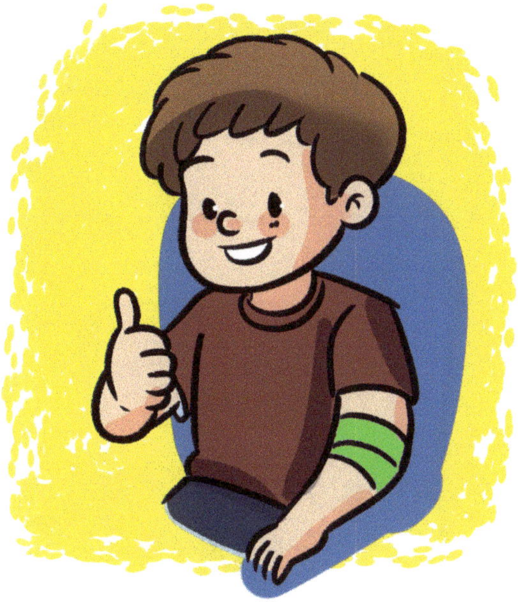

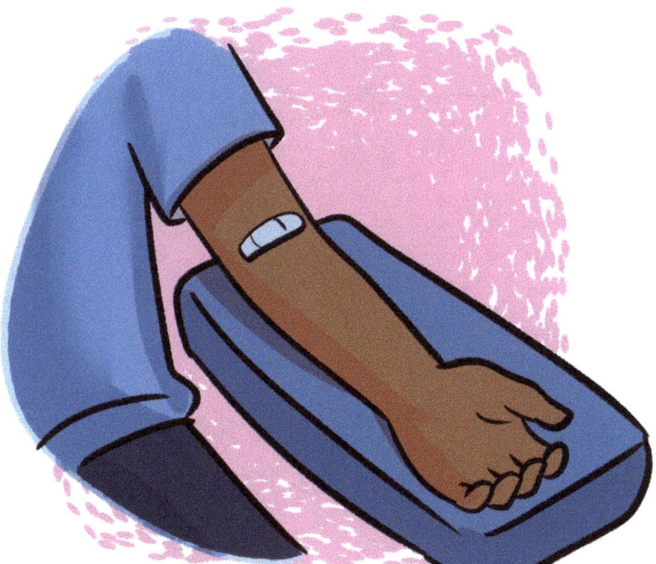

A colorful, stretchy wrap
or a small bandage
goes over the spot.

All done!

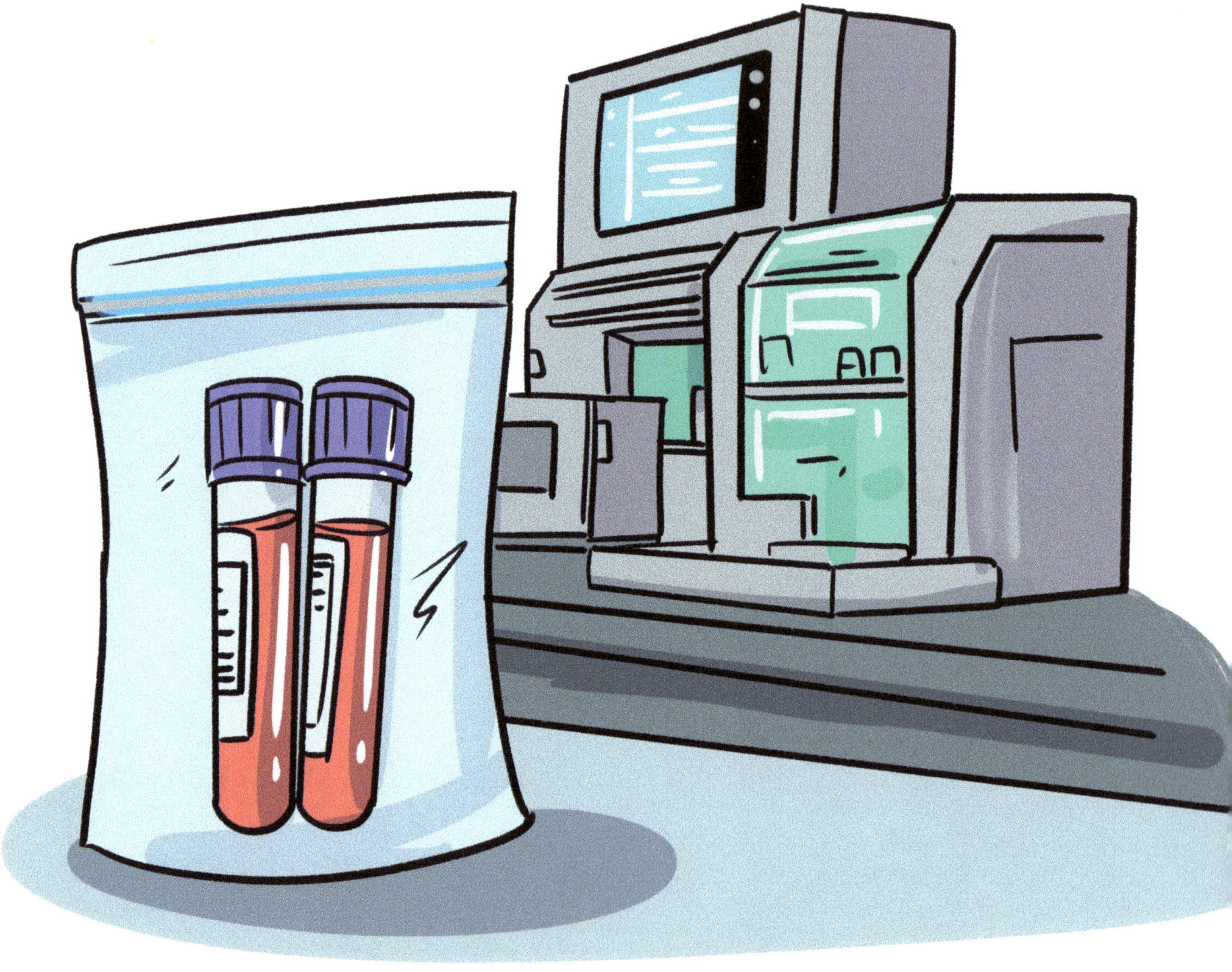

After the blood test, special machines and blood experts will look at your blood closely and carefully.

The blood test results help your doctor decide how to take the best care of you.

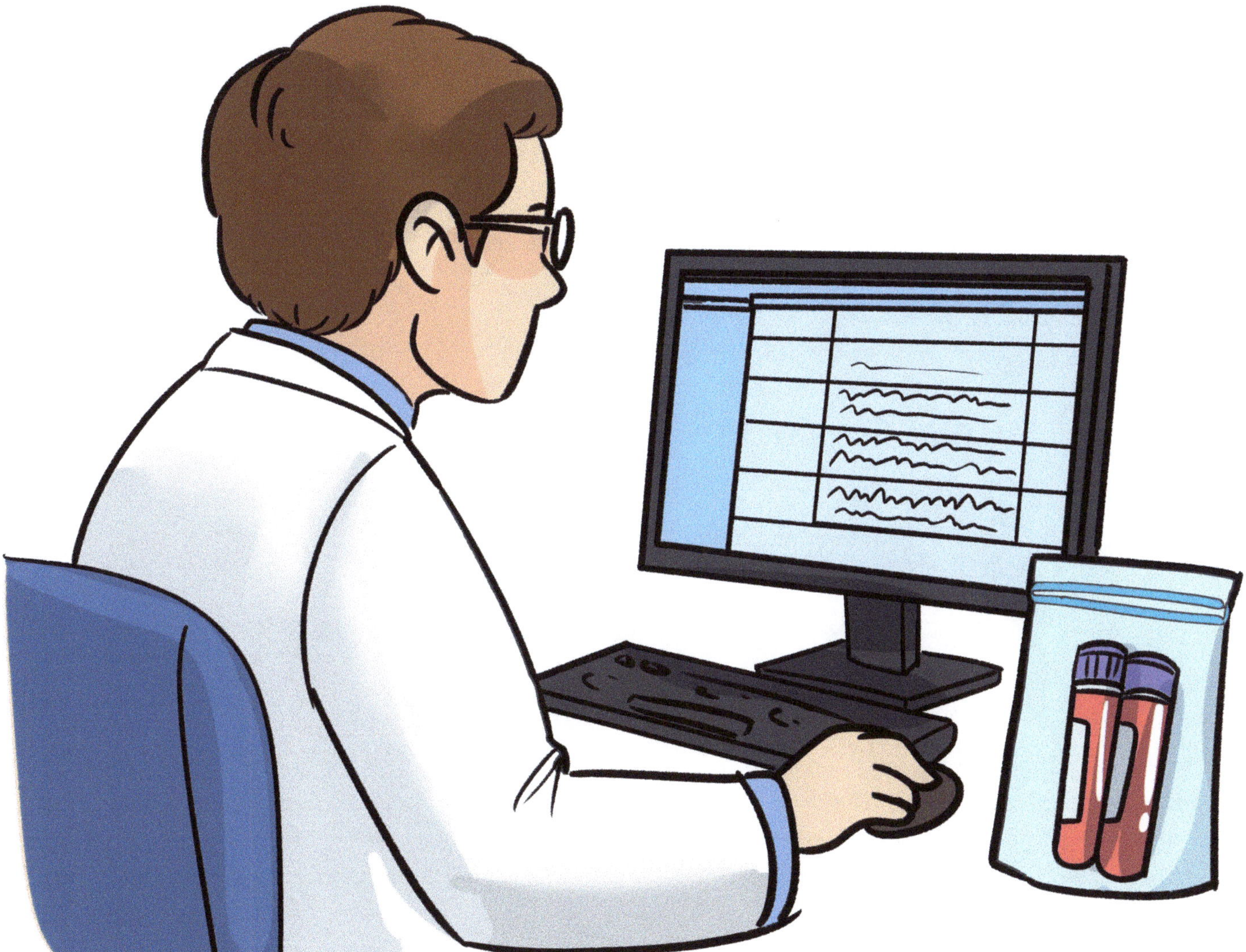

The spot may feel a little sore and may bruise, but that's normal and it goes away.

What would you like to do while the spot gets better?

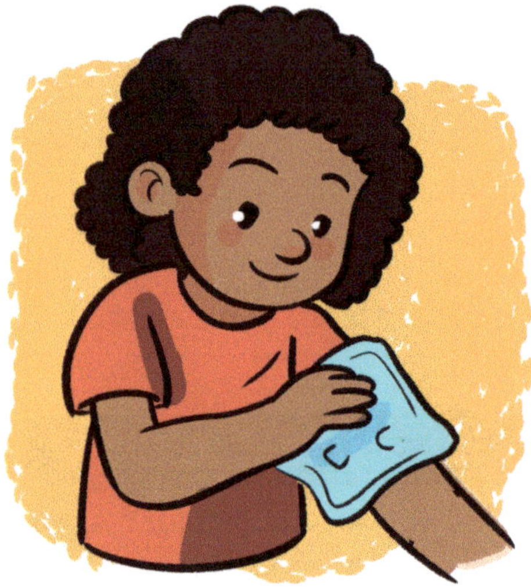

☐ Use an ice pack

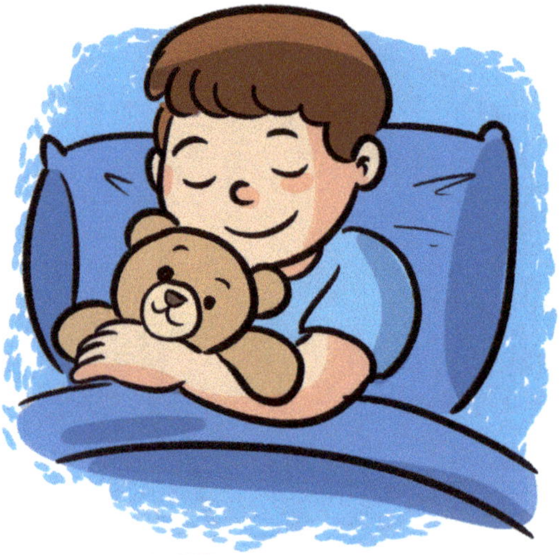

☐ Rest

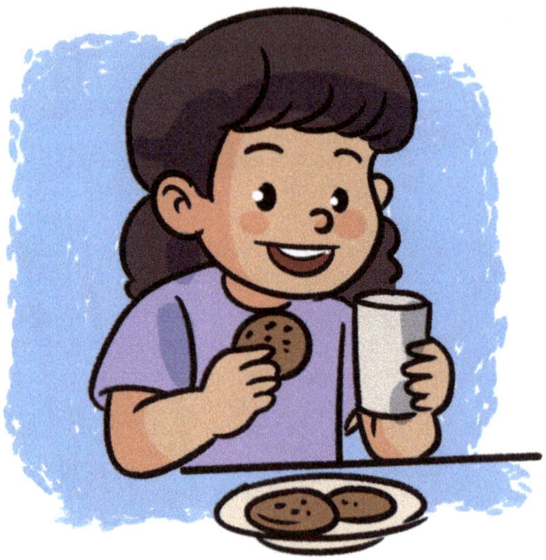

☐ Have a snack

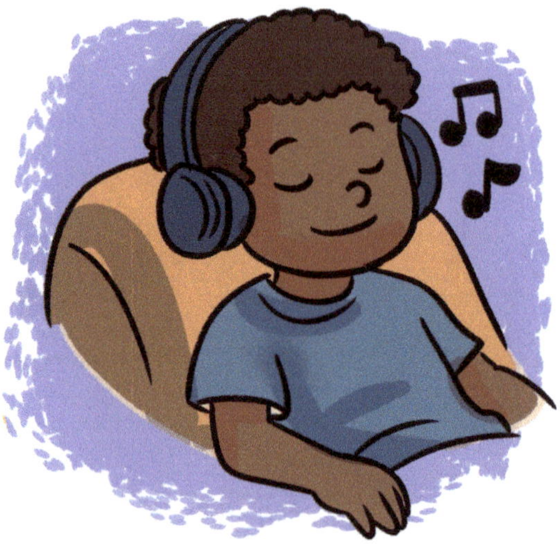

☐ Listen to music

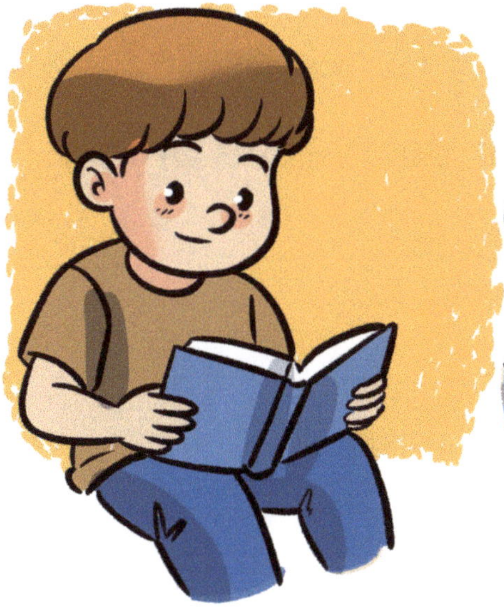

☐ Read

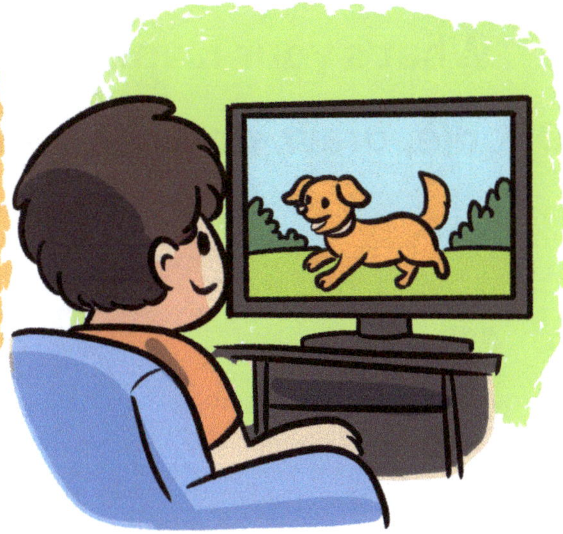

☐ Watch a movie

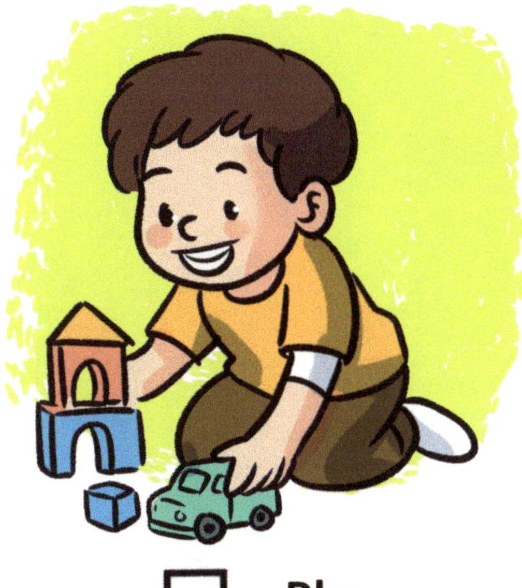

☐ Play

Most kids go right back to playing and their usual activities.

You are getting better every day!

What will you do after your blood test?

A party? A celebration?

What's your favorite way to celebrate?

Doodle, draw, or write your party plan below.

Speedy recovery!

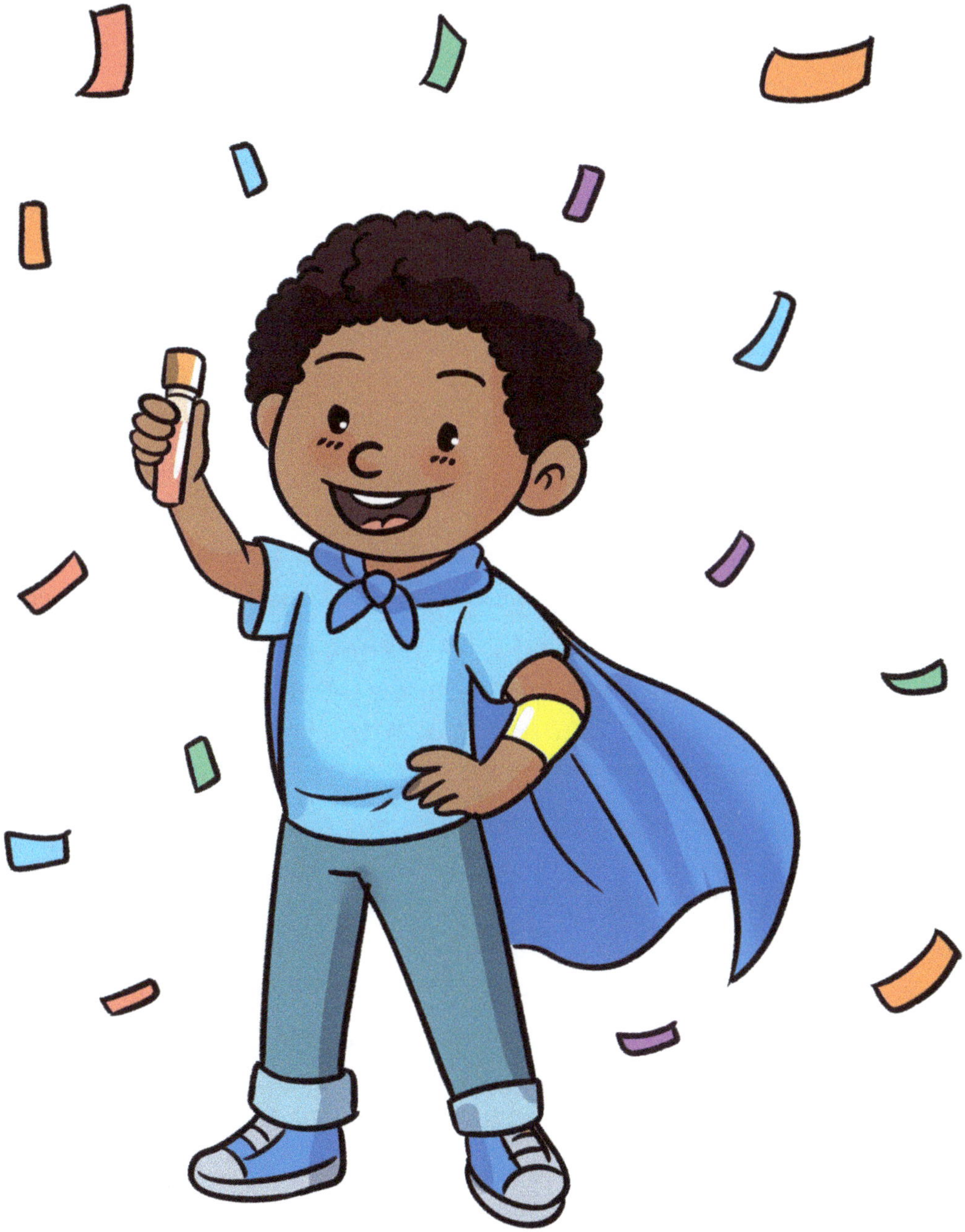

Notes for Parent/Guardian

• Encourage your little one to stay hydrated the day before their blood test to help the process go quicker and smoother. If your child is fluid-sensitive or has certain heart, lung, or kidney conditions, please speak with your child’s doctor first.

Disclaimer

Please note that the illustrations are not drawn to scale.

This book is written for informational, educational, and personal growth purposes and should not be used as a substitute for medical advice.

Please consult your child's doctor if they need medical attention and to ensure the information in this book pertains to your child's medical condition and needs. I cannot guarantee what your child experiences is exactly what is being discussed in this book.

The author and the publisher are not responsible, either directly or indirectly, for any damages, monetary losses, or reparations due to information in this book. By reading this book, the readers agree not to hold the author and the publisher responsible for any losses as a result of any errors, inaccuracies, or omissions in this book.

Please keep in mind that your child's experience depends on the location, the facility, their medical condition, and the healthcare team. Please use this book in conjunction with your child's doctor’s advice. Thank you.

Did this picture book help your child in some way?
If so, I would love to hear about it!

www.amazon.com/gp/product-review/B0H5NRV7PG

For other book titles, please visit:

www.fzwbooks.com

Connect with the author

email: books@fzwbooks.com
facebook/instagram: @FZWbooks

Books by the author

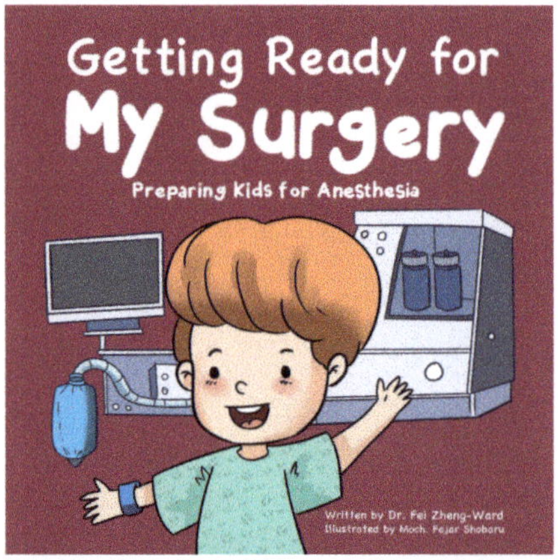

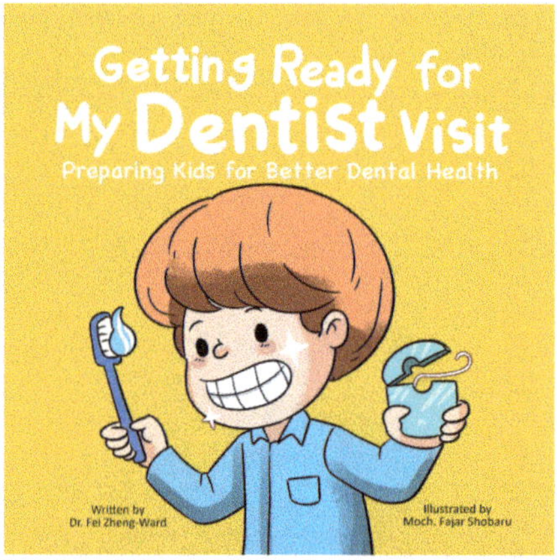

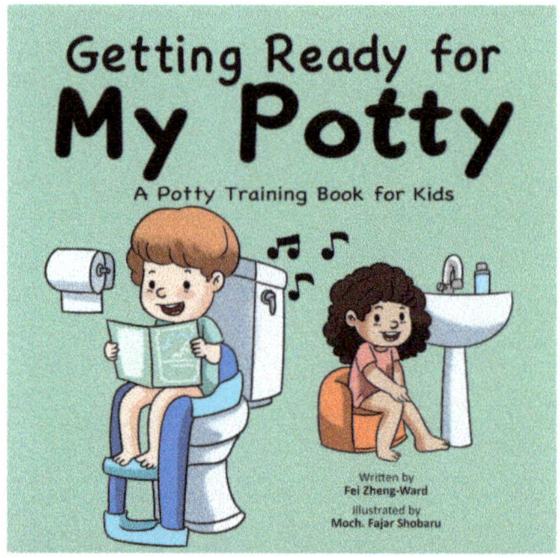

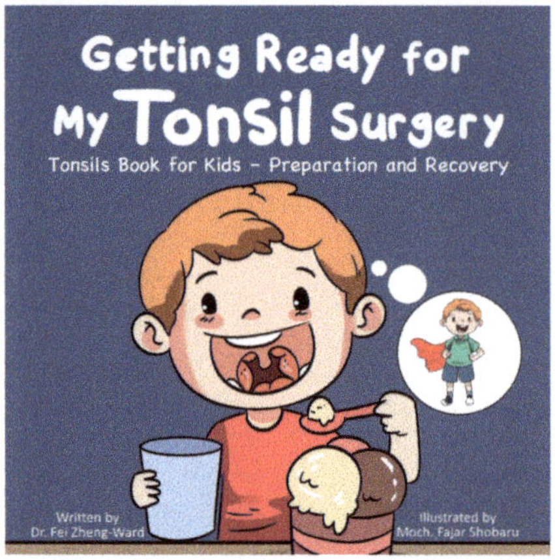

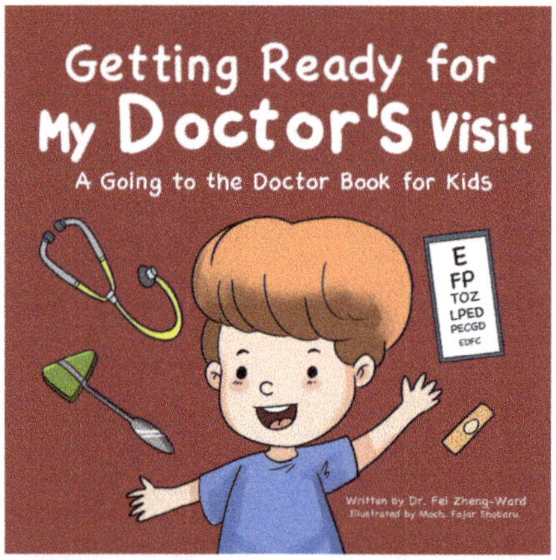

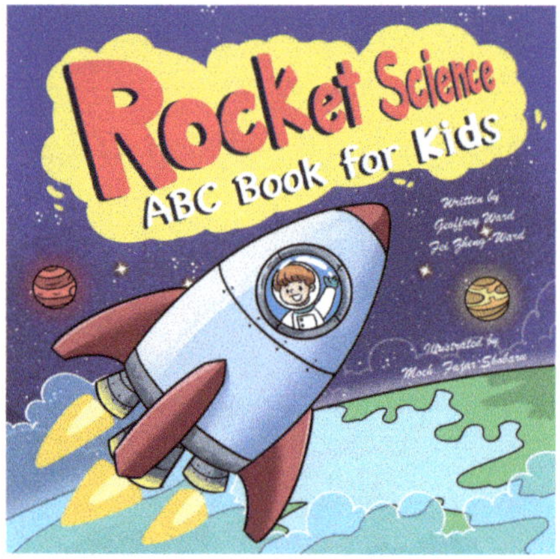

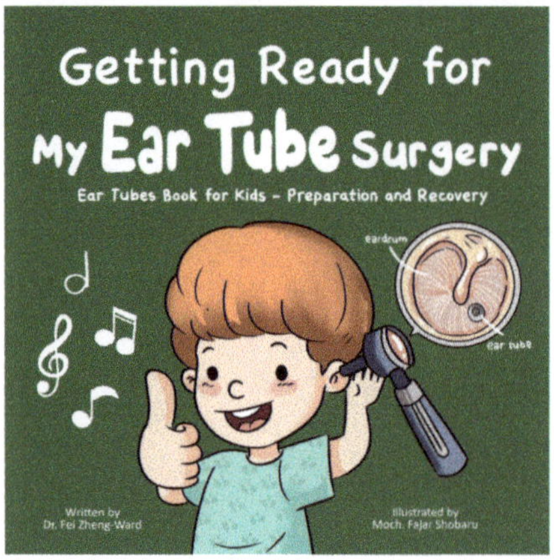

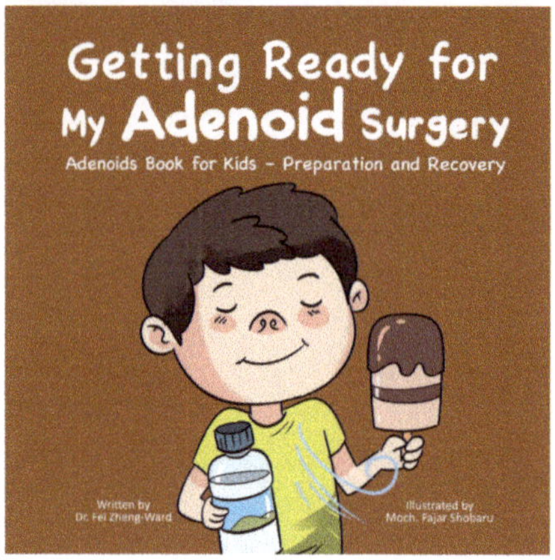

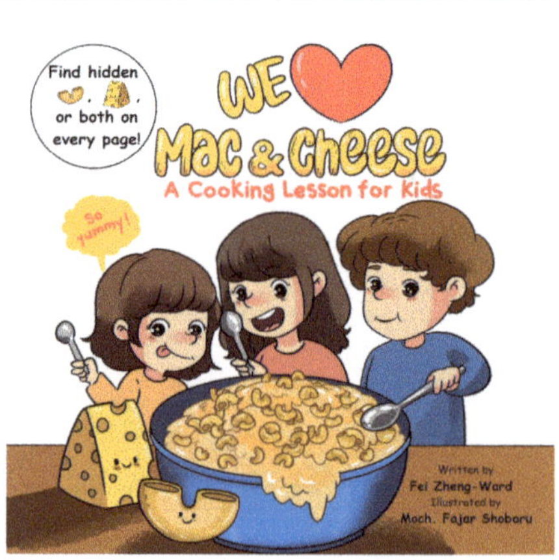

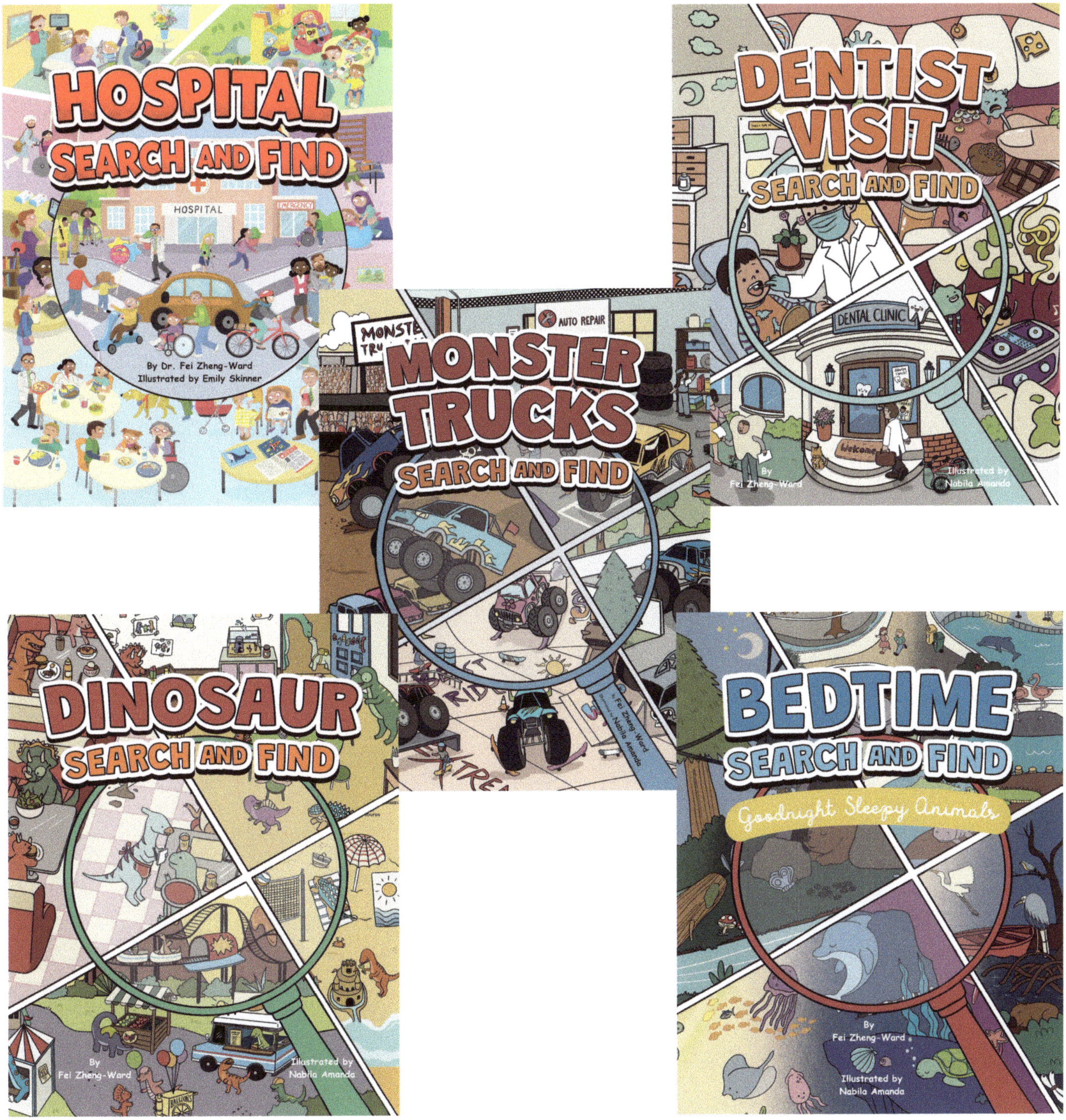
HOSPITAL
SEARCH AND FIND
HOSPITAL
EMERGENCY
By Dr. Fei Zheng-Ward
Illustrated by Emily Skinner
DENTIST VISIT
SEARCH AND FIND
DENTAL CLINIC
Welcome
By
Fei Zheng-Ward
Illustrated by
Nabila Amanda
MONSTER TRUCKS
SEARCH AND FIND
AUTO REPAIR
By Fei Zheng-Ward
Nabila Amanda
DINOSAUR
SEARCH AND FIND
By
Fei Zheng-Ward
Illustrated by
Nabila Amanda
BEDTIME
SEARCH AND FIND
Goodnight Sleepy Animals
By
Fei Zheng-Ward
Illustrated by
Nabila Amanda

www.ingramcontent.com/pod-product-compliance
Lightning Source LLC
LaVergne TN
LVHW070911210926
848482LV00017B/1052
* 9 7 9 8 8 9 3 1 8 2 0 1 9 *